M000099692

A Traveler's Guide to

Geriatrica©

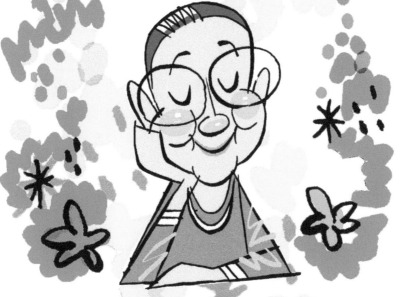

Marilyn Heins, MD

Illustrations by David Fitzsimmons

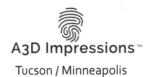

A3D Impressions™

Tucson / Minneapolis

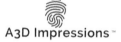

A3D Impressions™

First A3D Impressions Edition March 2020

Publisher's Cataloging-in-Publication Data

Names: Heins, Marilyn, 1930-, author |
Fitzsimmons, David, 1955-, illustrator.
Title: A traveler's guide to Geriatrica / by Marilyn Heins, MD;
illustrations by David Fitzsimmons.
Description: Tucson, AZ; Minneapolis, MN: A3D Impressions, 2020.
Identifiers: LCCN: 2020932430 | ISBN: 978-1-7344724-0-0 (pbk.) |
978-1-7344724-1-7 (eBook)
Subjects: LCSH Aging--Humor. | Old age--Humor. |
Aging--Psychological aspects. | Old age--Psychological aspects. |
Older people. | Older people--Health and hygiene. | Older people--Medical
care. | Older people--Care. | Retirement. | BISAC SELF-HELP / Aging |
FAMILY & RELATIONSHIPS /
Eldercare | HUMOR / Topic / Marriage & Family
Classification: LCC BF724.5 .H45 2020 |
DDC 155.671--dc23

Donn Poll, cover and book design

Dedication

This book is dedicated to all those who are traveling to or dwelling in the land of Geriatrica ...

... and to the two men in my life named Milton. The first Milton and I started the journey to Geriatrica. The second is helping me mightily along the way.

My heartfelt thanks

to the following people who helped me decide to write this book and shared their thoughts about aging. This book could not have been written without their help. They also supported me along my journey to Geriatrica ... whether they know it or not (and whether they are still with us or not).

Adele Barker
Nancy Bissell
Dr. Lynn Boysel
Ruby Buchsbaum
Helen Cohen*
Myra Dinnerstein
Lillian Fisher*
Dr. James Flores
Geraldine Forrer*
Milton Francis
Harold Fromm
Ann Gilkerson
Jeremy Glick
Hannah Glick
Dr. Rachel Glick
Jim Hays
Esther Heins*
Harold Heins*
John Hildebrand
Alexis Huicochea
June Hussey
Debbie Kornmiller
Judith Leet*

Dr. Dawn Lemcke
Jeb Lipson
Joshua Lipson
Mary Maher
Margie Matters
Larry and Rowena Matthews
Dr. Tamra Whiteley-Myers
Steven C. Neff
Dr. Gene Nightengale
Hester Obermann
Maria Parham
Dorothy Riley
Elouise Rusk
Elaine Rousseau
Tom Sanderson
Susan Seidl
Jane Swicegood
Ted* and Shirley Taubeneck
Sheila Tobias
Leslie Tolbert
Robert Weintraub
Angel Voyatzis
Sam Zelman*

I also want to thank my great-to-work with publishers Rick Wamer and Donn Poll at A3D Impressions.

Finally, I am thankful for and indebted to my beloved illustrator, Dave Fitzsimmons, who cleverly made this book as amusing and palatable as old age can be!

*deceased

TABLE OF CONTENTS

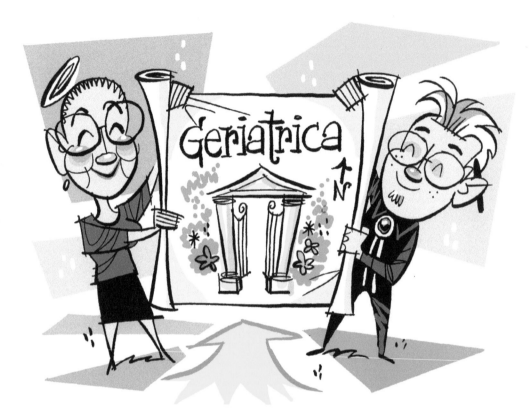

PREFACE

I am an immigrant to a new land where many, but not all, of my friends and relatives dwell.

No passport is needed. There is no border to cross. Sages tell us we live our lives one step at a time. One day, maybe without even realizing it, we step into Geriatrica.

Do I belong in Geriatrica? Absolutely! My driver's license affirms my age, my mirror confirms it. However, everything feels strange. Even though I have lived here long enough to speak Medicare I still feel like an immigrant sometimes.

Adjustment to any new land is arduous. This book will tell you what I have learned to help make your journey, or the journey of a loved one, easier. Maps included.

. . .

Let me introduce myself. I am a retired pediatrician and medical educator. I am 90 years old.

My personal story is that of a changing woman living in a changing world.

I was fortunate to be born into a family that valued education and achievement. My parents were of modest means but my mother worked as a commercial artist so I was able to attend college and medical school without the burden of student loans. My parents were also sending my sister to college at the same time and they spoke of having to return empty soda bottles for enough money to go to the movies.

In those days a woman's highest goal was motherhood, preceded, of course, by wifehood. In 1947 on our first day of college, the Dean told us we were there to become educated mothers for our children. I wanted to become a doctor so this was puzzling. Radcliffe never deterred me from pursuing my nontraditional goal, but I had to plow ahead alone because there were virtually no women role models.

I never thought of myself as a pioneer but in 1951, the year I entered medical school, only 394 women in the entire country did so (5.3 percent). In 2017 women represented 50.7 percent of the 21,338 matriculants. For the first time, the number of women enrolling in U.S. medical schools exceeded the number of men. If in 1951 I had known what a rare bird I was, I might have been too frightened to fly!

It was then perfectly legal to restrict the number of women entering medical school to five percent. In 1972 the Educational Equality Act made this illegal but it was not enforceable until 1979 because the College Athletic Association lobbied that football was a contact sport that women could not possibly play. Feminist activists sported bumper stickers that read, "Dancing is a contact sport. Football is a collision sport."

Medicine was definitely a man's world in those days. I look back at myself and those days with amazement. In my pre-feminist innocence and ignorance I accepted without question attitudes and treatments that today would lead to a lawsuit!

Third year medical students all were required to take a rotation in Obstetrics-Gynecology. Male students had an obstetrical on-call room in the hospital with four bunk beds and a bathroom with a shower. Students were on call around the clock and were expected to stay in the hospital.

I was assigned a cot in a closet-sized room, airless except for one window opening onto an air shaft shared by the quarters for research animals. I cursed the scientist using roosters in an experiment because no sooner had I fallen asleep after delivering a night's worth of babies than the roosters noticed the dawn.

Even worse than no sleep was the problem of keeping clean. Women students had to use the bathroom down the hall that did NOT have a shower. Desperate conditions call for desperate measures and I found the nerve to shoo all of the men out of their room and take over the shower.

The specialty of OB-GYN deals only with women, but enlightenment came slowly to this group. On the first day of our rotation the head of the department introduced the course saying, "With apologies to the women attending this lecture to become physicians, the function of young women is to have babies." Eighteen years later that remark somehow raised itself into my consciousness as I was hurrying to the hospital. I was so enraged if I saw that man in the street I might have kicked him!

My last year of medical school brought a moment of panic. I felt confident that I could be a doctor but suddenly had qualms about how to be a WOMAN DOCTOR. How do they manage to be doctors AND women? How do they have time for marriage? Children?

I boldly asked a married woman on the pediatrics faculty with one child and another on the way to invite me to her home. I was so glad to see her manage all this that I overlooked how tough it was to be pregnant, work all day, come home to mother a toddler, and entertain an anxious medical student! Only later would I understand the enormous challenge of juggling two lives.

I continued on my Pioneer Trail. I was the first woman to head a department at Detroit Receiving Hospital. Also the first woman to serve as an associate dean at two medical schools, as a vice dean at one, to chair the Group on Student Affairs of the Association of American Medical Colleges, and a committee of the American Hospital Association.

My husband was the REAL pioneer in our family. He allowed me to do my own thing and was a continuous source of encouragement and support. He also gave me the gift of mobility so that I could choose which job offer to accept. Thus I was the one who decided where we would live. I was accepted for a position at the University of Arizona College of Medicine and we moved to Tucson in 1979.

How did my family fare? One day when we were still in Michigan, my husband accused me of having my period weekly because I was so irritable on Tuesday after the Dean's meeting.

Why? I was the only woman in the room. When I said something it was often ignored but approved later when a man said it. I was ignored as were many other women in those days.

I am grateful that my children put up with me. I was the ONLY mother on the block who worked outside the home. A neighbor asked, "How can you bear to leave your adorable daughter at home all day with the colored help?" thereby crowding both racism and sexism in a 17-word question!

My daughter, then in medical school, joined me at dinner with two women physician colleagues while we reminisced about managing medicine and motherhood. My daughter spoke up, "You want to know what was the worst thing I remember?" My heart sank, here my deserved retribution comes! "In middle school I had to take the bus alone to go to the orthodontist and it was scary and I was the only kid in the waiting room whose mother wasn't there." We three women docs all offered much sympathy and understanding. Secretly I was relieved that this parenting sin was so venial!

My research at both medical schools looked into what I called Medicine and Motherhood: The Double Burden of Women.

Motherhood with a capital "M" started in the 17th century when kinship ties weakened and the nuclear family arose. Next came the concept of childhood. Industrialization separated the workplace from the home so fathers, nobly, entrusted the upbringing of their children to their wives.

Historian Gina Morantz-Sanchez spoke at a conference titled A Century of Women's Health I convened here during the University of Arizona's centennial. "Between 1750 and 1850 industrialization transformed the social meaning of gender roles. An ideology of domesticity glorified the separation of home and public life ... and the female qualities of nurturing, moral superiority and maternity."

The women's sphere was extolled by Catharine Beecher (born 1800) who glorified housekeeping as work assigned to women by nature and God. Women performed duties of infinite variety providing constant intellectual stimulation and good exercise. Like joining a health club today!

I wrote in 1997: "We must move rapidly to provide working parents with universal child care and parental leave. We need universal public preschool and schools that provide a menu of afterschool options."

"I have a vision for the future. In the 21st century, women will continue on the path to equal ACCESS to all education and career opportunities. Women will have increasing opportunities for ADVANCEMENT as the glass ceiling first cracks and then shatters. And there will be an ABATEMENT of the double burden carried by women who choose to have both children and a career."

I will leave it to the reader to answer the question, "Are we there yet?"

. . .

How did I become a writer? When I was in college my father suggested I offer the *Boston Globe* my services as a reporter of college news. I was already a reporter for the college weekly newspaper so it seemed a logical, if unlikely, job to apply for. To my surprise they hired me and paid me a dollar an inch.

Years later I thought it might be fun for me and helpful to parents to write a parenting column for the newspaper. The *Arizona Daily Star*, again to my surprise, agreed. This was in 1989. I am still at it but my focus has shifted to writing advice for the readers who, like me, dwell in Geriatrica.

I have the privilege of purpose in my life even though I am an old lady.

I still feel useful though I dwell in Geriatrica. For this I thank the *Arizona Daily Star* for publishing 1.1 million words of my columns, and also all my faithful readers.

YOUR MAP

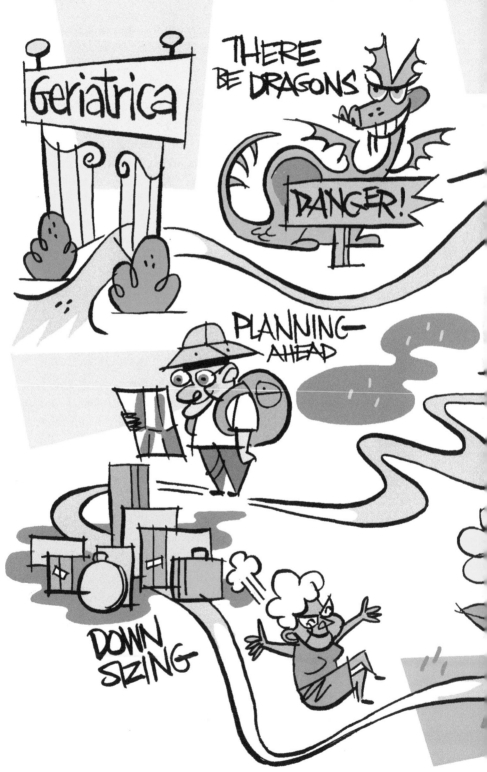

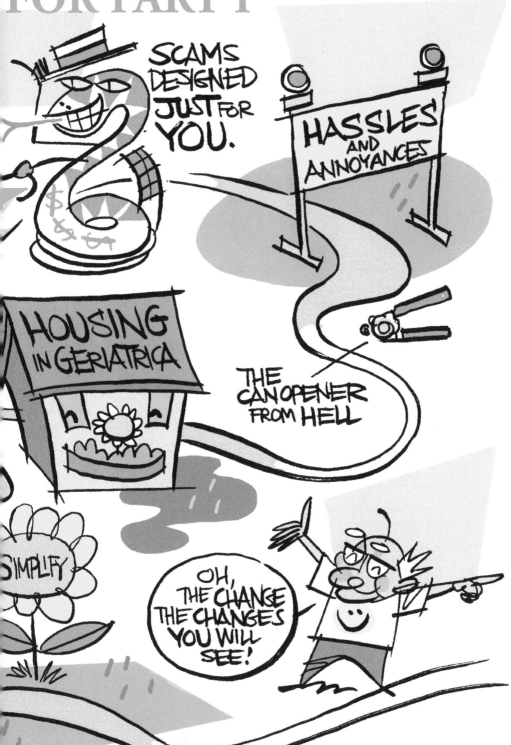

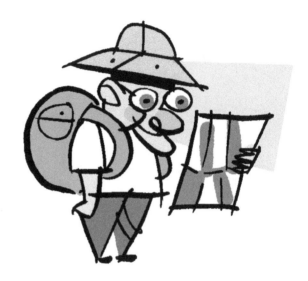

PART I INTRODUCTION

PREPARATION FOR YOUR JOURNEY

Guide books usually start out with information about the land and its people: topography, climate, population, language, industry. There are no geographical boundaries to Geriatrica as it is seamlessly interwoven with the Land of Youth and Middle Age. Thus when you step into Geriatrica much, if not most, of the landscape will be familiar to you.

However, the life you will lead in Geriatrica is ... or will seem to be ... very different.

Part I chapters will describe this new land, including the people who immigrated here before you, and the housing here. It will warn you about dangers and hassles and, like all good travel guides, will tell you how to plan for your adventures in this new land where you will live for the rest of your life.

Plan to live happily ever after. I did. And still do.

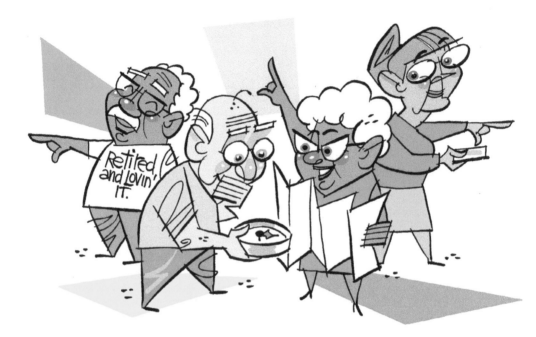

CHAPTER 1

A RECENT IMMIGRANT'S TRIP

I am an immigrant to Geriatrica, a land we old folks inhabit. I have a valid passport verifying I am now 90. But this land seems strange. What am I doing here? How did I get here?

The fact that I am writing this means I was blessed by Lady Luck. Lucky to be born to a family that, despite a very modest income, was committed to their children and could provide us with nurturing, health care, and education. Lucky to have good genes. Lucky to have a profession that enabled me to earn a living doing work I loved. Lucky to have my family and friends because we humans are herd mammals who need each other. Lucky I had the resources and stamina to visit 106 countries on this beautiful planet.

Who lives in my new land? Lots of folks at different parts of the aging spectrum. When we are in grade school we are pretty much like the other kids, similar in size and cognitive development (think back on your second grade class picture). As we age, we become more diverse. Some of us shrink a lot, some don't. We all have Medicare but some of us age well, some do not. Some of us have visible infirmities, some don't. We sag in different places.

Our role models for aging? My grandmother spent her last days dozing in a chair. My artist mother kept painting, despite failing eyesight, until a fall in her 90s. You will find many of today's citizens of Geriatrica are surprisingly active and vibrant. An astounding tidbit from census data: life expectancy at age 100 is 1.9 years for males and 2.5 years for females!

What do we know about the people who live in Geriatrica today? The number of people 65 and older is a whopping 52 million, 16 percent of the total population. Projection: this number will nearly double to 95 million, 23 percent by 2060! Wow!

According to the Population Reference Bureau, baby boomers (born between 1946 and 1964) " ... are reshaping America's older population."

"As they have passed through each major stage of life, baby boomers have brought both challenges and opportunities to the economy, infrastructure, and institutions."

We oldies are more ethnically and racially diverse. Life expectancy has increased from 68 years in 1950 to 78.6 years in 2017, because of the reduction of mortality in those over 65 thanks to Medicare and advances in medicine.

Challenges remain in our age group such as obesity, economic disparities, and Alzheimer's disease (predicted to rise from 5.8 million to 13.8 by 2050.) These will put stress on existing nursing facilities and Medicare expenditures.

Other challenges include the large number of childless elders. Childless couples are expected to be one of the fastest growing segments of the elderly population. Already 37 percent of women and 19 percent of men live alone.

It is estimated that there are many elderly people who have nobody.

These "geriatric orphans" have no spouse, adult children, other relatives, or support systems. Loneliness, like war, is not good for any living thing of any age.

On the plus side, we oldies spend less time in anger or worry than younger folks do. Despite infirmities we have a surprising optimism, less negativity about the world, and a better sense of well-being. Is older wiser? Yes. Our brains slow down but elderly folks make better decisions and recognize patterns better than younger ones do. Our memory for what we did yesterday may be shaky but we do well as a valuable memory bank about our past for the younger generation.

Erik Erikson, a psychologist and psychoanalyst, theorized about old age and lived to experience it. He described the stages of life and explained the developmental tasks of each. Erikson wrote that the last stage, Stage 8, begins at age 65 (he himself lived to be 92). The developmental task of the last stage is to attain what he called "wisdom." Old age brings inevitable losses. We become fragile in body, mind and spirit; we worry about dying and worry more about becoming dependent on others after a lifetime of being independent; we fear we will lose our purpose in life.

We seek wisdom by looking back on our lives, reviewing both our successes and our failures. We must try to forgive ourselves our trespasses and reach a place of peace. After all, why despair when we can do nothing about the past?

I recently did a review of my life. I went back over all the bad things I had done starting with what caused an embarrassing rebuke from my kindergarten teacher. (I was bratty then but I learned to be a good girl.) Before I reached middle age in my retrospective review of faults, I laughed out loud. My faults weren't the least bit original, darn it. I did make some mistakes in life that I regret. I am human and we all know Homo sapiens is not wise all the time. But I tried not to make the same mistake twice.

Wanting to balance my recollections, I wrote my obituary. This task gave me the chance to both remember my accomplishments and reminisce about all of those who helped me all along the way. I said many a silent thank you to those who are gone, like an aunt who died at 95. She gave me 500 dollars so I could afford my first trip to Europe. (She never let me pay her back, but I used her example to help others make a dream come true.)

What have I learned so far? It is a privilege to be in Geriatrica. Yes we must cope with losses but age can also bring us grace and dignity to face what is left. We must balance our lives and thoughts between the past and the present. Let's try to explain the pluses and minuses of aging to our family and friends. Only now do I understand how my aging mother must have felt when she ... a once energetic dynamo ... morphed into a fragile old lady. Let's stay connected to old friends and make new ones. Let's be as generous as we can to those who may need our time.

Let us be courageous. We are all descended from immigrants who had to be brave to make a new life for themselves in a strange place with a new language and new customs. If they could do it so can we.

Let us try to help others as best we can. Let's think about those who will one day become immigrants to Geriatrica. Though our own children are grown, let's think of the young children. They need to be educated so don't grumble about taxes. I heard Marian Wright Edelman speak at a conference many years ago. Her concluding remarks were. "The child you ignore today may be the one caring for you in a nursing home someday!"

Let us remember to keep our planet healthy. Earth is the only home any of us elderly folk will ever have. I hope my own footprint has been light and that our descendants will follow this path.

Two years before his death I asked my father what it was like to grow old. He replied, "Every day over 80 is pure velvet." I plan to cuddle up in each velvet day I have. What makes my day velvet is the privilege of still being somewhat useful to others. For this I thank my readers!

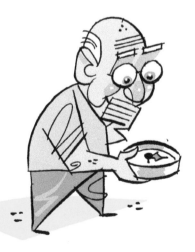

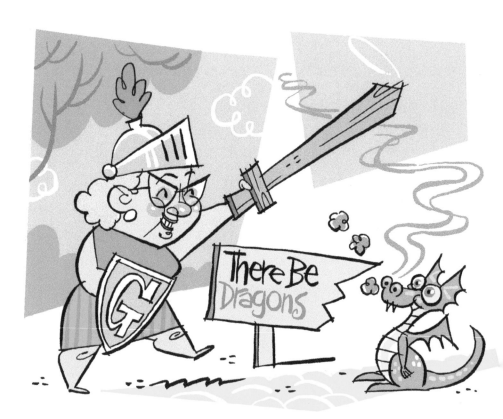

CHAPTER 2

THERE BE DRAGONS (DANGERS)

The expression "There be Dragons" meant dangers abound. It took many, many years to explore and map the entire earth. In medieval times mapmakers drew illustrations of dragons and other mythological creatures on uncharted areas of maps where nobody knew what was there because nobody had been there and returned. Ancient maps and globes reputedly labeled the unexplored sections "There be Dragons." (Actually Mr. Google just told me that only one globe, but no maps, had these words. Maps simply illustrated unexplored areas with scary creatures.) I will use the term because everybody knows the phrase meant entering such territory was scary and immigrating to any new land is scary.

When I traveled to a new country, I always read a travel guide first and took it in my carry-on to read on the plane. The guide always warned travelers about any dangers they might encounter. We do not have to worry if the water in Geriatrica is safe to drink but we are leaving our familiar land. You may scoff, "We left childhood to enter adolescence, didn't we? And we survived." True but the adolescent is full of energy. Those of us in Geriatrica aren't so peppy anymore.

BEING ALONE

When we hear the phrase " ... Until death do you part" at a wedding, no one, certainly not the bride or groom, thinks about the reality of their future. Statistically, barring some catastrophe that will get both their names in the news, one of them will be left behind when the other dies.

Being alone is hazardous to your health and well-being. We are a herd mammal and need others around us. Loneliness is a major risk factor for depression, with increased symptoms in both middle-aged and older adults. Social isolation is not healthy for anyone, but the elderly who may not have the energy to go out or may no longer be able to drive will feel this more keenly. (See Chapter 18.)

The Internet and telephone are links to the outside world but not all seniors are adept and many have trouble hearing. Being alone and becoming housebound can affect nutrition, taking medications, personal hygiene, and outlook on life.

Doctors worry about their patients who live alone and encourage them to seek and use available community services that, alas, are not available in all areas.

Savvy oldies who live alone recognize these dragons. Some have a pact with a neighbor who has a key to their house. They call each other every morning and if there is no answer they check the house. Some find a student who needs housing to live in. One woman I know persuaded a lady of her vintage to join her in her house and share expenses.

Women do better than men when they are alone because women are more likely to lunch together or engage in long, chatty phone calls. They are also better at keeping in touch with family.

FEELING USELESS

This feeling can be experienced even by those too young to live in Geriatrica. When men retire, they may feel they are no longer living a purposeful life. Buying a motor home or playing golf every day is pretty cool for a while. But this life style can also get old.

Women (and men too) feel purposeless when the youngest

child leaves home. The "empty nest syndrome" can cause an enormous sense of loss. The child-rearing role you have had for many years is over. Even if you were looking forward to the absence of dirty socks or pizza slices under the bed! I remember that the silence of the children's absence hurt my ears.

There is a cure for these feelings of uselessness. Get INVOLVED! Do volunteer work ... people are needed to help do everything from helping children learn how to read to feeding detained immigrants. Join church groups, take classes, start or join a book group, reach out to neighbors and friends.

Challenge yourself to fulfill old dreams. My mother decided to take piano lessons again in her late 60s because it helped her stiffening fingers. After retirement a friend finally had the time to practice and became a wonderful pianist. One aging physician I know took up guitar and even wrote some country songs. Another took up painting.

OUTLIVING RESOURCES

This is a scary dragon. Count on everything becoming costlier as we age and on living until you are well over 100. Plan ahead. (See Chapter 21.)

OUTLIVING CHILDREN

Losing a child is life's cruelest blow. When I was a medical student I noticed one of my octogenarian patients quietly crying in his hospital bed. Why was he crying? It was his son's birthday; the son had died 30 years before. I didn't know what else to say except I'm sorry but what popped out was, "Tell me about your son." I sat down at the bedside, he dried his tears, and was very eager to talk to me. When I had to leave he thanked me. I silently thanked the wise professor of medicine who taught me that the patient is first and foremost a person.

Some of us figure our children will always be in our lives. Let's all hope for this. Grandkids too! And great-grandkids as well!

COMMON FEARS WE EXPERIENCE

Elderly fears are inevitable and real. We fear the aging process itself. We fear the unknown future and losing our independence and autonomy, especially driving privileges. We fear we will run out of money or become dependent on our children.

We especially fear our own decline. Not driving can be mediated with Uber. Becoming immobile or demented do not have an Uber-like fix.

In heartfelt talks with friends in Geriatrica, there is a fear of horrible indignities that won't go away and will likely get worse. Incontinence, dementia, and helplessness top the list.

My personal approach is to hope for the best. Others tell me they will kill themselves before this happens. Alas, I see two problems with this escape route. You may not realize what is happening until it is too late to off yourself. Or you may botch the attempt and end up in worse shape than you were!

VULNERABILITY OF THE OLD

Oldies and children are always the most vulnerable. When there is a natural disaster such as an earthquake or flood, the very old and very young suffer. They are also the ones that suffer most in invasions or civil wars. We literally cannot run from danger and tend to hesitate, or not have the ability, to evacuate. Climate change also can be very hard on the elderly. As cities heat up and areas flood, we are often the hardest hit.

WHAT WE DO TO OURSELVES

The worst thing we can do to ourselves is become rigid in mind and spirit. It's only natural to cling to our old ways and habits. But age marches on as does time. If you have discovered a fountain of youth and found a way to reverse aging do let us know. If not try to enjoy, or at least tolerate, Geriatrica as most of us learn to do.

Another self-inflicted geriatric negativity is to cling to your past. Memories and reminiscences are good. The danger is when your past is a lifetime accumulation of "stuff" that you do not want to part with. The extreme version of this is hoarding ... never throwing away even a newspaper until the house is filled with trash. This is dangerous. Better to surround yourself with nice memories.

LIVING WITH LOSSES

As we grow old the loss pile gets bigger. There is a simple formula: longevity equals losses. Loss of our youth, loss of our loved ones, loss of our abilities. If we are lucky our body and brain deteriorate slowly but nobody gets to Geriatrica without experiencing loss. Let us hope our losses are balanced with gains of wisdom, insight, serenity, and acceptance of what we are today and have become.

I once read "The basis of a person's life is hope. Where there is hope there is life and not the other way around. When there is no hope for the future, there is no power for the present." Thank you, Dr. Ken Olson, for these wise words.

Fellow Geriatricans: Hope your own future! I hope your own journey has been long, the source of wonderful memories, and that you now can live in peace. Que sera, sera. (I'm sure you all remember Doris Day!)

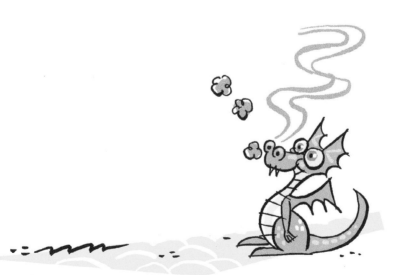

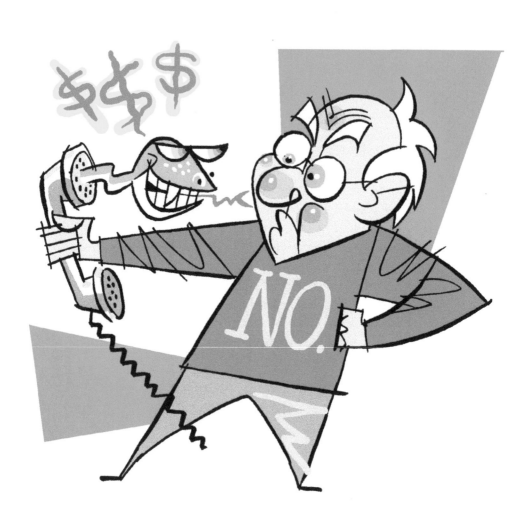

CHAPTER 3

SCAMS DESIGNED JUST FOR YOU!

As if we elderfolks didn't have enough to worry about like the high cost of prescription medications, we are being specifically targeted by smooth-talking telephone scam artists.

Family emergency scams are common and can enrich the scammer by defrauding the grandparents. Posing as a relative or friend of someone you know like a grandchild, the scammer tells a story asking for emergency funds to help with a dire emergency. Send money for bail, a hospital bill, or having to leave a foreign country! Send it quick! Or else!

The story can sound plausible because the scammers are very good at what they do. The tale they tell is scary and always demands ultra-fast action. I got one of these calls several years ago from someone purporting to be my grandson. ("Grandma this is your grandson. I am desperate! I need your help!"). Because I have three grandsons I asked which grandson are you. He did not identify himself so I hung up. Was I sure it was a scam? Yes. Was I worried maybe it was not a scam? Yes, but I used the powers of reason and common sense to calm me down.

There are other scams besides the Family Emergency Scam. I get multiple phone calls from scammers saying they are the Internal Revenue Service or Social Security. If I was stupid enough to pick up a call from a number I did not recognize I hang up immediately muttering curse words I didn't even know I had in my vocabulary! Microsoft calls are mildly amusing. We are told if we don't respond immediately all our data will disappear. Our data remains intact but the calls keep coming. Why? It is cheap and easy to make zillions of calls a day.

The numbers of calls are staggering, According to *Consumer Reports* these monsters who blithely disturb our tranquility and train of thought in the privacy of our own home can make over 3000 calls per second. Or *147 million* calls per day!

Why are the elderly targeted? We are usually at home. Some of us lack technology smarts. Many of us live alone and being alone makes any scary thing scarier. Fear escalates when we are isolated. Those of us with mild cognitive impairment or dementia may be easily fooled.

What can we do? 1. Verify the "emergency." 2. Familiarize yourself with the tricks scammers use. 3. Report a scam you have responded to so that the FTC (Federal Trade Commission) and state attorney general will have the information.

How do we verify? Don't panic! That is what the SOBs want you to do. Verify the person's identity by calmly asking things no stranger could answer. Call the supposed family member. If you are worried and alone, call a friend or family member even if the caller told you not to tell anybody. **Never send money by wire or a check by overnight delivery.**

Tricks used to fool you are amazingly successful and only one or two responses will make the scammer's day. Scammers know you are elderly and can easily and quickly use social network sites to get enough information about a family member to fool you. If you get suspicious, they may ask you to talk to an accomplice who is said to be a lawyer or police officer. They play on your emotions and may even impersonate your grandchild as my scammer did. They swear you to secrecy so you don't ask someone you trust what you should do. They insist you wire the money immediately before it is too late.

Use common sense. I knew my grandson would identify himself. Any time you are asked to send a large sum of money quickly, resist! Hanging up is the best way to deal with these tyrants. If it really was a hospital they will keep calling. Call a child or friend to talk about this scary event. When we talk about something scary it helps us calm down.

Family emergency scams are the worst. They scare the vulnerable into acting quickly to send money. But there are other calls invading the castle we call our home. Thirty-nine percent of robocalls are scams and 17 percent are telemarketing. The rest are alerts to tomorrow's doctor appointment or a payment. I tabulated the number of robocalls I got at home in one day. It was 20, all scams or telemarketing! I just hung up ... Microsoft was calling!

I try to rely on Caller ID and do not answer any unknown person or number. But these clever callers "spoof" us by using a local number or even a name. When we answer it is a lowlife telling us we won something or that they want to give us money if we do what they ask. The most recent abomination: the phone rings and the caller I.D. was me! Don't pick up or the robo caller knows you are a live victim. Remind yourselves that a caller we need to talk to ... a relative, doctor, lawyer ... will call us back. But darn it, I **really** resent being disturbed by a ringing phone.

Cell phones no longer protect us from robocalls. Because my family and friends know I prefer to be called on my landline, there can be 10 or more unwanted calls on my cell and no "real" calls.

Another way thieves prey on the elderly is identity theft. If you leave a letter containing a check or a credit card bill in your mail box, this can be highjacked. I take such envelopes to a mail box or post office. Always check your bank and credit card statements.

Tyranny has had many faces in history. Kings and their subjects, slave owners and their human property, factory owners and their underpaid, overworked workers. Tyranny is power over people, stronger humans over weaker ones.

Today we live a new age of tyranny by technology. It happened so quickly and can morph so fast that we the people have no recourse. The French, American, and Spanish revolutions were won by armies. Factory owners were challenged with labor unions.

How will we all unite to fight the Technology Revolution? And could any of us give up technology that makes our old lives easier and brings us a grandchild's smile via FaceTime?

What is the answer? Regulation can and should help. Be sure your land line and cell phone are on the Do Not Call Registry. It is far from perfect but does help. There is also new technology on the horizon that will be able to authenticate phone numbers using a digital signature.

Robocalls are the largest source of FTC complaints today. Several categories of robocalls are currently legal. These include political parties and charities, for example, as well as information calls from doctors and pharmacies. I politely (mostly) say, "I do not support a cause or buy goods from any organization or business if I am disturbed at home. I only respond to a mail or email request." Note that some spoofed calls are legal. A women's shelter that does not want an abuser to know a victim's location is one example.

Survey data: 15 percent of people say they or a loved one had been reached by and scammed by a scammer. All of these, plus the rest of us who are annoyed every day by such calls, should support and demand regulations.

The elderly, who especially need telephone communication in case of an emergency, should join the fight. NO MORE SCAM CALLS, NO MORE ROBOCALLS! We have lived long enough to earn the right to peace and quiet in our own homes!

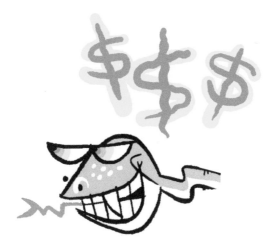

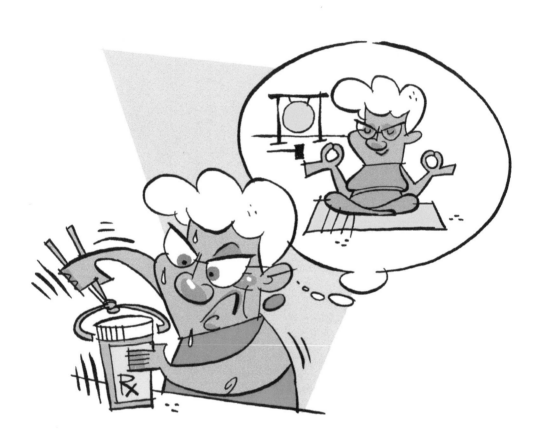

CHAPTER 4

HASSLES AND ANNOYANCES

A recent trip to the drugstore led to five hassles. Mr. Google informs me that a hassle is an irritating inconvenience and that the word may have derived from combining haggle and tussle. My definition is an irritating inconvenience that one not only struggles with but cannot stop from recurring.

My hassles? All items from the drugstore I had trouble opening. A shower cap and cuticle remover were each locked inside cardboard my ancient fingers could not pull apart. I had to get the heavy-duty scissors I keep in the kitchen to use with recalcitrant food packages. I then had to return the scissors to the kitchen as on some occasions they are the only thing between me and starvation when the food comes in a box.

To open Lip Shimmer and something called Master Concealer I first needed to get a pointy scissors to pry open some sticky tape. This was followed by a trip to the first aid kit for a hemostat (a surgical clamp used to control bleeding that I have had since I was in pediatric practice and I retired nearly 30 years ago.) The hemostat finally clamped on a bit of the tape so I could remove it. "Tear tape?" I call it Tears Tape ... tears of frustration.

The fifth hassle was opening a new medication prescribed for me. It required a trip to the garage to get the right size pliers that would open the bottle without destroying the lid. But I had to wait until stronger hands came home because I couldn't get the ancient pliers to work.

I know products are tested before they go on the market. I respectfully request that products be tested not only on toddlers to ensure they CANNOT open a bottle of medication that could be harmful but also on us seniors to make sure we CAN open a medication we need. "Push down with palm while turning." What is Plan B if the lid does not budge?

Why does newsprint seem so anorectic these days? Skinny paper has taken over the world. Refolding a newspaper is close to impossible. And both entire "sections" within a newspaper section, or even a single page, can slip out to the floor when one tries to turn a page. Paper in magazines and catalogues frustrates me because it can be so thin pages stick together and have to be peeled apart.

It is a hassle for me to deal with my computer that insists on the now or later installation of upgrades and apps. Computers love to update themselves but I hate it. If my screen does not look exactly as it did yesterday, I may have an anxiety attack. To be honest I can sometimes figure out by myself what the screen now tells me. But often I need to call my computer guru for an installation tutorial. This is especially hassle-y when I have a deadline.

Other hassles? Pop-up ads on the screen when I want to read an article online. Commercials on TV that are unbearably loud as well as horrifically repetitive. Cable listings of zillions of channels not in alphabetical order. Network TV shows that stop every few minutes for commercial breaks and are disturbing to me because I am so attuned to cinema that my nerves are jangled by a six-minute drama.

Mailboxes (both those at the end of the driveway and in my computer) stuffed with junk. People who don't pick up their dog's poop. Huge boxes sent at Christmas time filled with more food than two people can possibly eat.

Music lovers at a concert who cough and THEN think to unwrap a cough drop. Concertgoers who hum along or move in or out of time with the music.

Movie lovers who crunch nonstop through a two-hour movie. Movie theaters that play previews so loud I must cover my ears, hearing aids and all. Movie theaters and other public buildings that are air-conditioned to such a low temperature my teeth chatter and I must carry a sweater when it is 102 in the shade outside.

Voice mail robot telephone calls that repeat so quickly my ancient fingers can't press delete in time so I have to listen to the damn thing again. Especially maddening when there are subsequent calls that I do want to hear waiting for me to delete this one.

Telephone calls answered with a lecture. "You have reached the office of Dr. Smith. If this is a medical emergency please hang up and dial 911. If you know your party's extension dial it now. If you wish to make an appointment, good luck! (Sorry, I made that one up!) If you wish to make an appointment press 1. If you wish to cancel an appointment press 2. If you prefer to not wait on the line press 3 to leave your name and number. You will be called back by a patient representative sometime between now and next Christmas." I better stop this or I will get really cranky.

Telephone calls I make answered by a person whose voice is too soft for me to hear even with my expensive hearing aids and special telephone. Or whose accent is hard for me to understand. I now say upfront, "I am hard of hearing, can you please speak up or get someone else I can speak with?" I also try to prepare for the call beforehand so I have all I need at hand.

Where are you now, Lily Tomlin, telephone operator par excellence? I really need to hear your strong voice and ask you to connect me with the person I need to speak with now.

Fact: I cannot stop hassles. They are entrenched in modern society. Are we oldies affected more than young folks? Maybe, because of the myriad "infirmities of age." Are they more common than in the past? Seems so, because we are so attached to and dependent on screens and telephones. Do they ever go away? Yes, they can vanish or be replaced. I remember holding a baby in one arm and a fork in the other when the doorbell rang. At least we no longer have a Fuller Brush Man to disturb us.

Maybe, just maybe, I will find antidotes to hassles. Deep

breathing can help. I find if I stop trying to do a task and just walk around the house or take a "time out" my agitation lessens.

When I was a busy young mother with two toddlers and a full time job, I learned a lot from my children. One day when I hung up the phone, distressed by hearing about the severe illness of my elderly grandfather, my daughter said, "Mommy, why are you mad at me?" She interpreted my frown as anger. I went to the mirror and saw she was right. I did look angry.

That taught me to take a quick peek in the mirror when I am upset. The mirror tells me there are better ways to look and feel than angry or upset. I may smile at myself, stick my tongue out, or mimic an opera singer belting out an aria. This nonsense helps me find perspective.

Other things like a reading break or doing a few clues on a crossword puzzle help my agitation fade. When I go back to the hassle task it somehow seems easier.

I use a similar technique when I have misplaced something. If I go from place to place frantically trying to remember where I left an object, it often eludes me. Instead I sit down, close my eyes, and try to access in my subconscious mind what I did with the object. The subconscious mind is a huge memory bank that stores everything but does not always like to release the information. I pretend I am a very quiet, very lazy detective trying to solve the case. Amazing! It works most of the time. When it doesn't work, the location of the permanently lost object may forever remain a mystery.

I am also learning to trust my subconscious mind, ancient as it is. While thinking of something else entirely, the thought of my health insurance cards popped up. I was already disrobed on my way to the shower but I stopped to put my insurance cards in my purse as I had a doctor's appointment later in the day. Seize the moment or else!

I recently read an article about how nature can help young children with behavior problems. A mother wrote to ask me about her six-year old son with ADHD (Attention Deficit Hyperactivity Disorder). I suggested nature walks, collecting rocks, and planting a garden to teach patience.

My HA (Hassle Agitation) also responds to being outdoors. Just walking down to the mailbox may do it, but sitting on the patio and looking at the clouds is sure to work. It's a nice place to wait for Strong Hands to come home and rescue me.

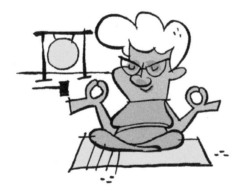

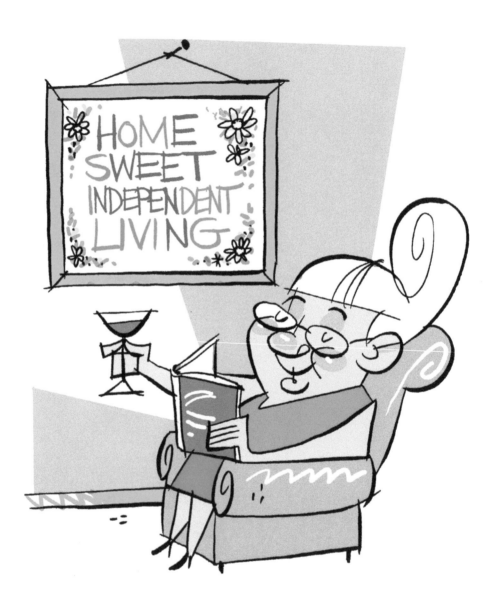

CHAPTER 5

HOUSING IN GERIATRICA

WHAT'S AVAILABLE HERE?

Where do people in Geriatrica live? What is available for those who are no longer able to live alone?

In days of old, families took care of aging kin at home until they died or became so feeble that they needed nursing home care. Nursing homes, like hospitals then, consisted of wards with several or many patients. Care was often suboptimal. Wards could be smelly and little attempt was made to provide stimulation or comfort, just minimum care of bedridden patients.

Out-of-home care for the elderly was started in the early 19th century by religious groups and fraternal organizations. We have come a long way in the development and expansion of care for the elderly. Now there are about 2000 Continuing Care Retirement Communities in the US. These CCRCs are designed to offer a continuum of aging care needs ... independent living, assisted living, skilled nursing care, and memory care ... all in one facility. This is a growth industry necessary to meet the needs of our aging population.

The continuum approach to aging is designed to accommodate the changing needs of the elderly. Advantages include being able to stay in one location for the remainder of your life, living with less anxiety about your future, being with your own age group, having activities on site, and avoiding becoming dependent on your children. Disadvantages include costs and added costs for additional care needed as you age, giving up your "nest," and downsizing which means parting with some of the treasured possessions that you, like all the rest of us, have accumulated.

Some definitions for those who have put off thinking about aging and for the children of aging parents. CCRCs are described above. Independent living means just that. You can live independently because you can care for yourself. Assisted Living provides care like showering and dressing when you can no longer do this safely by yourself. Memory Care enables patients with dementia to live safely. A Skilled Nursing facility provides a high level of care (IVs, breathing tubes for example). This is the place you go to for rehabilitation after you have been released from the hospital, and, hopefully, will be able to go home soon. Or the place you go when Assisted Living care is not sufficient to meet your needs.

In Anne Tyler's novel, *Ladder of Years,* an aging grandfather describes Senior City, the name of his high-rise retirement home. "We're organized on the vertical. Feebler we get, higher up we live ... strikes me as symbolic." He goes on to say he pictures life there as a ladder " ... a ladder on playground slides, a ladder of years where you climb, you fall over the top, and others move up."

Another model of Independent Living is a complex for a community of people ... there is an age limit on the lower side, usually 62 ... who live in apartments or small houses. Dining, public spaces for events, a gym, and other amenities are provided on site. A nurse is often available for the care of minor health problems and there is a connection to physicians. Maintenance of the units is provided as well as lectures, concerts, and other communal activities.

I liken this to a hotel with concierge services 24/7. Instead of trying to find a plumber to fix a broken toilet you simply call the front desk. Health emergency like a fall? Call the front desk.

This model does not guarantee continuing care. Such care is available on site or nearby but there will be additional costs to cover the additional care. Some facilities do not have any skilled nursing care so you would have to move if you needed it.

Warning: There are two kinds of continuing care. One guarantees care for life after you have paid a large sum for the independent quarters you live in. The other does not have a complete "ladder of years." I have heard horror stories about those who assumed they would be cared for in their senior facility forever but were tossed out because they became too ill or enfeebled to stay. Be sure you ask about and understand the policy before you sign on the dotted line.

Other models offer different combinations. For example, Independent Living and Assisted Living are provided in the same units. The big advantage is you don't have to move when you need more care. Some private homes are licensed to care for a small number of patients who cannot live alone or take care of themselves.

I became familiar with some of the various senior facilities when family members or friends were planning a move. I saw many of the local facilities when visiting friends there. One couple I had known for many years needed my help to make their decision, choose a facility, and move in. I watched them both ascend the "ladder of years" as chronic illness in one worsened, and a stroke felled the other.

MAKING THE DECISION

Pediatricians are about as far removed from geriatricians or gerontologists as one can get! However, because of my own advancing age, I have had to think about my future. Becoming familiar with what is available is step one. Step two is making the decision.

This decision is not an easy one. But I never heard anyone say, "We should have waited longer!" I did hear, "I didn't realize how much running a home on my own was stressing me." "I wish I had faced what loneliness was doing to me. I kept trying to suck it up!"

The challenge of aging is to accept our old selves. We ain't what we used to be! And we will never again be that person because age and time each go in only one direction. Age goes up, the time left to us goes down. Two more ladder metaphors!

I once wrote that the decision should be made 1) Sooner rather than later. 2) Early enough so you can move as a couple. 3) Early enough so YOU make the decision of where you want to spend the rest of your life, not your children! 4) Early enough after being widowed so you do not spiral downward. A widower told me that he felt alive again after the move helped reverse his debilitating loneliness.

I have known couples that were not at the same rung of the ladder. One was independent, while the other needed more care. One couple told me that they were grateful the facility enabled them to stay together. A man I talked to confessed he would never have survived living alone in the house after his wife was gone. Another man said that, when his wife developed dementia, he was grateful they had made the move. He could visit her every day by just walking over to the Memory Care unit. She was in a safe place. And he had friends on site to help him deal with his grief.

A dear friend said she felt very fortunate to be able to manage her failing husband in their independent living apartment with part-time help for showering and getting him to the doctor. "Because I didn't have to cook or shop, I had the strength to just be with my beloved. We held hands and watched old sitcoms or movies. Friends dropped in. One lady brought her dog to visit every day."

Here is a question I answered that points out possibilities and pitfalls.

"I am 83 years old and live alone. My husband is dead and all my children live far away, one in Europe. My oldest son lives 1800 miles away and is very successful in his business. He has asked me to move to his town. He will build an addition on his house for me or find me a condo nearby. He already told me he would finance my move. I don't want to move away from my friends and the home my husband and I built almost 40 years ago. I am being pressured and I don't know what to do."

I answered, "First of all you are fortunate to have a son able to make this offer. In addition to providing a place to live he is committing himself to always care for you. (I suggest you thank your son profusely ... many elders I know would like to adopt him!) If you are able to care for yourself, explain your feelings about staying in your home and ask if he will provide funds to ensure your home is safe for you. I would also tell your son you might accept his offer in the future. Reserve the right to change your mind because a few years from now you may be very happy to sit nodding by the fire in the cozy addition to your son's home. And this will relieve your son of the burden of flying 1800 miles if you fall ill."

The woman who wrote to me described a pretty common dilemma these days ... an elderly parent living alone with children living far away. This is a result of the many societal changes we have witnessed in our lifetime. People are living longer and family members are often widely scattered geographically.

I urge all residents of, or future immigrants to, Geriatrica, especially the ones living alone, to gather information about senior facilities. Look online. Ask your friends, they are probably thinking about their future too. Visit facilities together. Have lunch there to get a sense of the ambience. Talk to the residents.

Such visits have two purposes. 1) To show you what contemporary facilities are like and how different they are from the nursing homes of old. 2) To decide which one best suits you in terms of location, amenities, and cost.

In summary, let's look at what the housing options are for those in Geriatrica. We can age in place, in our own home. We can age in place after moving to smaller living quarters in our own town. Relocate to a house or apartment where a child lives. Move to one of the senior facilities located where we live, or where a child lives.

The Centers for Disease Control and Prevention defines aging in place as, "The ability to live in one's own home and community safely, independently, and comfortably, regardless of age, income, or ability level."

This sounds ideal. "We don't have to leave our home!" But

physical and cognitive declines will likely require hiring more help and perhaps house modifications like wheelchair ramps. Thus, the resources we counted on for our old age may not be enough. This is especially true of those in the middle since those at the top can afford it and there are some government resources for those at the bottom.

In the Utopian future architects might help by designing houses suitable for aging in place, but not alone. Several wings, each with a bedroom and bath for privacy, located around a central living area and kitchen. Congenial individuals can agree to live there together and share expenses for household, drivers, and caregivers if necessary. My imagination does not extend far enough to figure out what to do when one sharer dies or congeniality ends.

MAKING YOUR DECISION

The factors that influence the housing decision we must make are age, physical and cognitive health, financial resources, and how we feel about these options.

We make decisions about our future based on the person we are now and what we can do now. There is a pitfall here. As we continue to age we are likely to do less, go out and entertain less, and watch our friends dwindle away. Try to imagine such possibilities as you think about your options.

Acceptance of our new selves in Geriatrica is not easy. Fast forwarding to what our future selves may become is near impossible. First of all we live in, and are rooted in, the present. UCLA's Hal. E. Hershfield reports that more than half of adults questioned said they did not think about what their lives might be like 30 years hence. In a brain imaging study, subjects were asked to think about their future selves. The way the brain lights up then is quite similar to how the brain reacts when we are asked to think about other people today. In other words, it's darn near impossible to picture our future selves.

Nonetheless we citizens of Geriatrica should try to accept who we are right now and who we may become in the future. Looking in the mirror, and acknowledging the fewer things I can do now compared with what I could do five years ago, worked for me!

MY DECISION

I am an elderly parent with no children living nearby. One lives on the West Coast, one on the East Coast, one in the Midwest and one in the South. Our family spans four time zones!

I have already decided not to age in place. First of all, I do not have the potential resources I might need to provide caregivers when I grow older. And I know I will not want to make a move at that time. Nor would I likely have the physical or emotional strength to do so. Most important, I want to be in a community to avoid loneliness as I begin to have less energy to drive to a class at the university.

And I definitely do not want to leave Tucson, a community I have lived in for 40 years and love for its beauties, the cultural opportunities, and especially for my many friends. I have planted deep roots here.

I do not plan to move closer to one of my children. Their careers and retirement plans mean they are as likely to move as to stay "in place." Thus, relocation is not in my cards.

I have chosen to move to an independent living community. There you can stay in your apartment and read poetry or you can play tennis with a new friend. You can make a meal in your kitchen (small kitchen with a big microwave) or go downstairs for a meal.

You are living with a community of people like you. But you make the choice. I feel like being alone today to finish reading the great book I started. Or I feel like seeing and being with people today so I'm going downstairs to the lecture.

My thoughts about the move? After a lifetime of running a house (much of the time also working at a busy career) I will be very happy to relinquish domestic duties! Planning for meals, shopping, cooking, cleanup all are time-consuming. And at this point in time, time is my most precious commodity.

My personal decision to move from my much beloved home of 40 years has been made. I will reside in an independent living facility now being built.

I look forward to being part of a new community of like-aged and like-minded people. I will rejoice to surrender the chores of domesticity and have time to write, read, stream movies, listen to music, or just sit in a rocking chair. (Note to self: buy a rocking chair.)

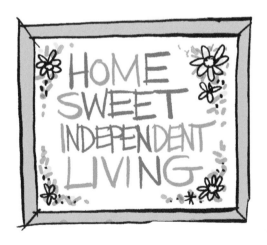

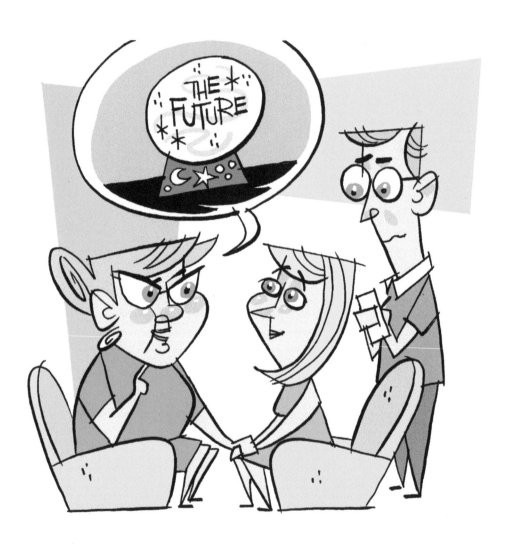

CHAPTER 6

PLANNING AHEAD FOR YOUR TRIP

PLANNING AHEAD FOR YOUR TRIP

Just like an adolescent we have to make decisions about our future.

The tasks of adolescence are to become emancipated from one's parents, figure out how to make a living, and find a mate.

In Geriatrica our tasks are, or should be, not becoming a burden to our children, having enough money to survive on even if we live to be 100 plus, and making sure we will always have people to interact with.

A TALE OF TWO WOMEN

My mother was an educated and talented woman born in 1908, 12 years before women could vote. She was an artist who drew department store goods for newspaper ads before photography and digital art. Her passion was painting flowers and her botanical art is in several museums.

My father died when Mother was 87. She lived alone in her art-filled house with the beautiful garden she planted and tended. She drove and continued painting and gardening until she fell and broke her hip. She stayed in her home, utilizing round-the-clock help, for more than 10 years. My sister lived 20 miles through Boston traffic away. I lived across the country, a day-long plane ride away.

My mother got her wish to age in her home. She had two devoted caregivers. Though she could not afford it, she had a generous grandson who could. It sounds idyllic and in the beginning it was. Family, friends, and neighbors visited. The family gathered at her home to celebrate birthdays and holidays. I called her every day. We chatted about many things and relived many memories.

But as she aged in place, she outlived all her friends. She became frail, reluctant to leave the house, and lived her last years in loneliness though my sister and I visited as often as we could.

There was nothing her daughters could do to cajole or convince Mom to move closer to one of us (I actually had plans drawn up for an attached guest house) or to a senior facility. First she said she needed her studio. When she could no longer paint, "I will NEVER leave my house!" became her mantra, frequently repeated.

My sister had the "geographical burden" which she bore with much grace and devotion until she herself became ill. I lived across the country but called to speak not only to my mother but also to her caregivers. I managed the "medical stuff" as best I could from afar. I visited as often as I could (my husband was ill and they both died the same year ... the summer and winter of my discontent).

Mother's garden became neglected, the house filled with magazines and much other "stuff" she would not throw away. She refused to give away my father's clothes. I spent a whole day in the basement going through many volumes of my father's engineering journals to find the ones in which he had a paper or was cited. Sweaty and dusty I handed her those, which she cried over, and told her that the other journals were already in trash bags. When I left, one of her caregivers was ordered to put them all back!

My Aunt Helen made a different choice. When her husband died after 60 years of marriage, my aunt was devastated and frightened. She often called me sobbing and I assumed this was grief. After several such calls I realized that, in addition to her grief, she feared being alone and had become too scared to drive.

Her son and loving daughter-in-law found a nearby senior facility they all liked and helped her downsize, move, and figure out what to put where in her new little apartment. She blossomed there and made many friends. And enjoyed the talks and concerts on site for many years. I called her every day too, and still miss hearing the voices of both ladies that were so dear to me.

"REVERSE PARENTING"

"Reverse parenting" is my term for situations when aging parents can no longer care for themselves and adult children must assume care. This always feels like upside-down parenting and it may be difficult or even impossible.

A question from the adult child of elderly parents. "How can I get my parents who are almost 90 to dispose of their many items stacked in boxes in every nook and cranny in their house and garage? I am not talking about clutter, it is much worse than that. My children and I will do the work but we have to know what is valuable and what they want to keep."

My answer dealt with the dangers of such hoarding (fire, falling over one of these boxes) and suggested ways to coax Mom and Dad (one box or room at a time, work together at speed parents can tolerate, make helping the parents a festive occasion where the generations laugh together about a 1940 wedding dress and you promise to keep the dress for your granddaughter's wedding).

I have looked at this "... from both sides now" to quote Joni Mitchell's old song. I was the child of aging parents and now I am an aging parent. Both roles can be tough.

I worried and fretted over my mother living alone. My children already worry about me as I will likely become less able to be independent. What is the answer? How do we coax or convince aging parents to listen? Can we? Should we?

Whether I write about young children or old folks, safety is my first concern. Yes, we want our toddlers to develop autonomy but we must prevent them from running into the street. We want our parents to remain and feel independent for as long as possible, but not at the expense of their safety and well-being.

I advise adult children and parents talk about these issues before they happen although this didn't work with my mother. My mother was able to age in place in her home of many years. Most of us, including me, do not have the means to do so. Or do not want to. I know 1) I will likely become less active as longevity proceeds. 2) Being alone is hazardous to your health.

Both parents and children should familiarize themselves with this issue. First become familiar with the types of senior facilities that are available today. (See Chapter 5.) When you visit a facility take a look at Assisted Living and Memory Care. You may be surprised how pleasant and attractive these facilities can be today. Plus it's a good idea to visit both before you need either.

Many of us have bad memories of visiting a relative in a nursing home (my parents would never let me visit my beloved grandfather so I imagined he was in a horrible dungeon). There is an enormous difference between nursing homes then and the senior facilities available now.

Over the years I visited several friends and my aunt in independent living facilities in both Tucson and Boston. I saw cozy individual apartments all furnished differently, pleasant dining rooms, and public space for events. There was socialization instead of a sense of living in "solitary" which happens to many of us when we can no longer drive.

What about those like my own mother who resist or even sabotage you? Do the best you can. I installed fire alarms in her house, kept in close contact with her doctors and caregivers (I loved these women and we still keep in touch) and worried an awful lot. I also called my mother and her caregivers every day and always left a number where I could be reached.

One woman I knew took her mother, who was failing and repeatedly falling, out to lunch. She then drove Mom to her new home in Assisted Living. I do not recommend such draconian action but I recognize and must point out that sometimes the children do have to act.

Information about such facilities is available from community agencies like Pima Council on Aging ... a Tucson treasure. Talk to others who experience similar frustrations with aging parents. Visit facilities to be prepared to answer your parents' questions (and plan for your own future).

"THE TALK"

Some aging parents do not talk about illness or death. They may feel their children do not need to know about all this until the end. They may be protecting the children from such matters, just as they protected you in the past. If the family is only together on holidays, celebration is in order, not gloom.

Children of aging parents, you may have to start the ball rolling. I advise you to talk to your parents long before they are in advanced old age. These days we hear dreadful language in movies and on cable TV. People talk and read about sex without batting an eyelash as my mother used to say. But death? The last taboo.

Don't be squeamish. Have "The Talk" about end of life decisions. Familiarize yourself with the issues. Long before your parents need it. Aging parents, if your kids don't bring it up you should. Problems can best be resolved with knowledge and dialogue. Not silence and avoidance.

Having "The Talk" is essential. It can be as difficult as having that earlier talk about sexuality but take a deep breath and talk about options.

Talking about topics like health, mental status, and money may make you uncomfortable. Not talking about these issues until there is a crisis is silly. It's like not talking to your kids about sexuality until pregnancy occurs.

LEGAL MATTERS

Everyone should have a signed will, Power of Attorney to make decisions for you if you become incapacitated, and a Durable Power of Attorney and Living Will so your end of life decisions are spelled out carefully and completely. I also signed a "Five Wishes" document available from Casa de la Luz Hospice that enabled me to spell out the specifics of what I do and do not want done when I am unable to care for myself or tell others what I want done (play music from my CD collection) or not done (religious observances).

Without these documents the decision between safety and autonomy may have to be decided in court. You will have to present evidence to the judge that your parent can no longer care for self or make decisions.

Your children need to have copies of all these documents. Ideally, you and your children have already talked about matters and they know where all the paperwork is.

Your children should know your health information. List all your doctors and their contact information, your medications with dosages and times you take them. Carry this list in your wallet.

In addition, your children should have information about your resources: lawyer, financial advisor, accountant, banks, insurance, etc.

For those who have no children you can leave your money to any person or charity you like. But the person you choose to make health care decisions for you when you cannot should be someone you know who agrees with your decisions and will carry them out.

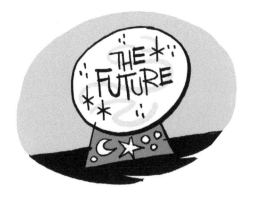

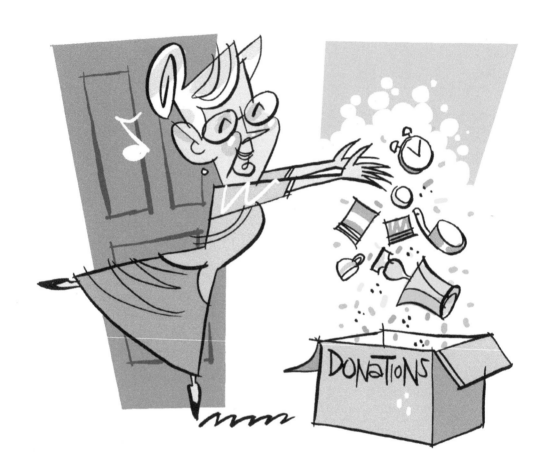

CHAPTER 7

DOWNSIZING

Look around you. I bet you are surrounded, or even engulfed by, "stuff."

Even those of us who do not fall in the hoarder category have more things than we need or use.

What happens to our stuff over time? 1) It accumulates, no it mysteriously multiplies. 2) It is transmogrified into clutter. 2) We trip over it. 3) Organizing it takes time which is the most precious thing we have at our age. 4) We fear our heirs may be burdened by sorting it all out (or fighting over who gets what). 5) We wonder how it will be possible to downsize when we want to ... a smaller house, senior living, or a move to be closer to our children.

How do we even start to downsize all this stuff?

Pediatricians like me are really into prevention. We want to immunize all our patients so they do not get childhood diseases like we did. We give anticipatory guidance to parents so they will childproof the house before the child learns to crawl.

Here is a new word: elderproof. Like childproofing, elderproofing our home and life starts with prevention.

Maybe the Medicare Card of the future should come with a document that reads "Buy Less! It saves the planet and your sanity!" It took me a long time to realize I did not need most things that I was urged to buy in newspapers, periodicals, TV commercials, and side bars on the Internet. I found I could travel to a distant land and not buy a single souvenir. I brought home only memories and cell phone photos.

Everybody our age should have a will. It should make clear who gets what.

I took photos of my entire house with a written key to what is valuable or was a legacy from an ancestor. This folder is with my will and executor letter.

Whenever a child or grandchild visited recently, I asked each one to tell me what he or she might want. I wrote it down. I also suggested things, "Grandpa would have wanted you to have this." It was amazing that the children wanted different things so there was no conflict. I hear too many sad stories of fights between the heirs after Mom and Dad are gone.

It is our task to deal with all of our stuff. Even if you intend to age at home downsizing is important. Not only for safety reasons but to "declutter" your brain.

At this writing I am planning a move to an independent living facility so I am right in the middle of downsizing. I have lived in my house for 40 years. It is filled with the usual suspects: furniture and memorabilia from a lifetime of living and traveling. The walls are covered with paintings done by my mother, a world class botanical artist, and framed memorabilia.

Surfaces are covered with framed photographs of loved ones and many knick-knacks. This cute word is defined as "small, worthless objects." Yes, they are small but worthless? A child's first attempt at pottery is precious to a Grandma.

The antique furniture and botanical paintings have been assigned to my children. I am giving away some things now. My biggest problems are the many, many books and other stuff made of paper.

I shudder to think of how many trees were cut down so I could collect this stuff. But in my defense, some of the books go way back to my childhood. And that was a very long time ago. Disclosure: Every year or so I reread *Little Women,* the first grownup book I read. I treasure some books that belonged to my parents and even my grandparents.

I never counted my books but I have nine large bookcases plus four walls of shelves. One grandchild wants my art books. Another wants all my books on women in medicine. Addendum added to my executor letter? Check.

I have zillions of books on parenting and on feminism. I called Casa de Los Niños, a local agency that deals with children and parents and those books will be donated when I move. The University of Arizona Gender and Womens Studies will take the many books dealing with feminism and women's struggle for equity.

What about the rest? I will take my poetry collection so I can keep rereading poetry. And *Little Women* of course. Plus a few favorites and a bunch of "horizontal books." Books that I have already read are vertical as if shelved in a library, and alphabetical by topic ... more or less. Books I have bought but not yet read are horizontal. I will have to decide which of those I still want to read and therefore move with me. I also have a Kindle, so far used only for travel as I love having a real book in my hands, but it will save some trees in the future.

What about the rest? Just this year I needed to know a simple fact. When did the Rogers and Hammerstein musical *Carousel* open on Broadway? I saw the great musical and was trying to remember the year so I could figure out when I met a friend in New York City.

I went to the book case that holds my theatre books and hefted a thick book from the bottom shelf, a book on Broadway plays and musicals. I could hardly lift or hold the darned thing. My hands were aching but I found out that *Carousel* premiered in 1945. As I struggled to bend down and put this heavy book back in its place, I realized there was another, less painful way. All I had to do was Google "Year *Carousel* opened on Broadway." Book Epiphany: no one needs to take any reference books with them when planning a downsizing move!

My CD cabinet will come with us as will many of my books on music because I simply cannot live without them. I also have a big collection of opera librettos that at the moment I cannot part with. I bought the almost crumbling *Tosca* libretto when I heard Maria Callas at the old Metropolitan Opera house. I was then studying medicine in New York City. Seats were very expensive, even in those days, but if you waited in a long line you could buy a standing room ticket. I was an impoverished med student in the days before student loans. Standing for the entire opera meant sore feet but it was worth it.

Paper takes up a lot of space in my house, and probably yours. We all save something! Examples: newspaper clippings, special letters from family and friends, old magazines, letters, recipes, wrapping paper, catalogues, tax returns, etc. I have a file cabinet in my office that has things I need to keep like financial records and bequeathal stuff. It also has memorabilia like family trees from both sides of the family that relatives researched and sent to us. After I weed out unnecessary folders, this file cabinet will come with us when we move.

In my garage are two tall, ugly, black metal file cabinets with a total of 10 file drawers. They contain many years' worth of clippings and reprints I used in my teaching and writing. The files are being carefully reviewed from my downsizer's viewpoint. Most have been recycled. A few autographed papers plus the papers I wrote or the talks I gave will go into a box. Even a committed downsizer will take a carton or two to take to her new, smaller place!

Clothes? Have you ever known a woman who had too few clothes? I have more than a few because I still wear some things that are well over 20 years old. Have I mentioned I hate shopping? Confession: I am guilty of helping to kill retail and I know there is no privacy in a world ruled by the Internet. But the convenience of online shopping is addicting!

Nonetheless my goal is to try everything on (a few each day) and only take the clothes I need and still want. Moving to an apartment by definition means a home with fewer and smaller closets.

Photographs? My computer guru has digitized many boxes of slides and albums of prints which were divided into two categories: children and other relatives including some faded pics taken before the ancestors left Europe and zillions of travel photos taken on our many trips. I will take the digital versions with me but also take some precious framed and unframed prints. The rest will go to my daughter who will decide which to take or distribute.

Grandchildren are captivated by photos of their mom or dad in diapers. My daughter will likely keep many of these. This is how "Stuff" continues unto the generations! We all go from being children to parents to becoming history!

Knick-knacks from trips, the little do-dads that one brings back, will not move with us but I will put my favorites together and take photos of the batches. Those little things that school children make in school and bring home are too precious to discard. What I plan to do is send them to the child or grandchild who made them. Shh ... it's a surprise!

Dishes and other kitchen stuff will be the most downsized. Future entertaining will take place in restaurants or consist of a glass of wine and some nuts to nibble on in our new home. I am designing my life, or rather redesigning it, to align with Geriatrica. Domesticity no longer interests me. Been there, done that. Besides it takes up too much time, a commodity that is "downsizing" as I write.

The cookware I plan to take will be very minimalist. "Pot and pan" will replace "pots and pans" in my new home. I look forward to a pretty empty fridge and cupboards. Actually, I plan to emulate Old Mother Hubbard.

Recipes, some of which are hand written by my mother or by me as my grandmother dictated, will go to my daughter. Complicated recipes á la Julia Child and cook books will be offered to friends or given away.

Not all furniture can or should go with us. Pieces will be out of scale or ready for the yard sale after 40 years of use. I look critically at each piece of furniture and plan to take only comfy pieces. The opposite of clutter is minimalism and I sort of look forward to it!

There will be bumps on the downsizing road. I hope I will be able to deal with them. Moving at any age ranks pretty high on the Holmes/Rahe scale of stressors. Saying goodbye to my house after 40 wonderful years and giving up my gorgeous mountain view will not be easy. But I am looking forward to moving into a community of other folks like me. Folks who have much less to do in terms of domestic chores and more time to write and read and watch the sunsets.

PS I just received an email from a very wise and knowledgeable lady who wrote that there is a better word to use than downsizing. At our age when we need less stuff to worry about but more time and leisure, the word is "rightsizing." I totally agree!

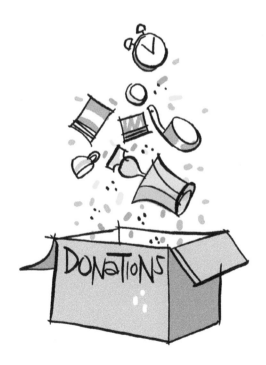

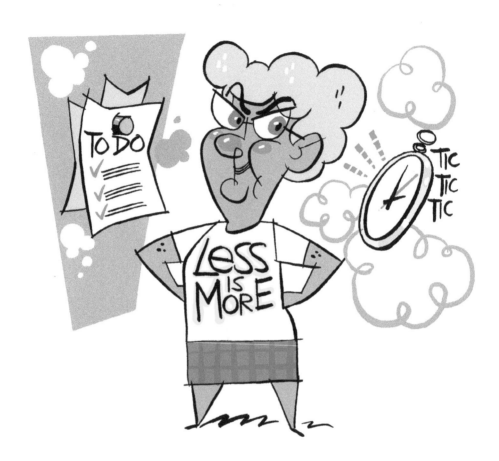

CHAPTER 8

SIMPLIFY! SIMPLIFY! SIMPLIFY!

As we age, our lives and our brains as well as our homes get cluttered. How can we declutter ourselves?

Every now and then I look back at each consecutive year starting with my first memory. Even bad or sad memories are useful. Some failures and painful losses end up on the plus side of my life ledger because I survived them. Odd how reflection on time lived is somehow soothing even if, or perhaps because, it brings tears.

I observe my own aging as objectively as one can and I talk to friends in my decade and beyond. I have come to believe that we all experience struggles with the seesaw of aging. We are high in the air to be faring as well as we do, but we drop way down when we realize new losses have arrived or are nigh.

I lack the wisdom to tell others or myself how to deal with this emotional seesaw. But I will share what I try to do.

Balance is important. I strive, not always successfully, to balance my day between doing and being. This involves planning ahead as well as taking my energy temperature at the time.

One advanced nonagenarian told me she had renewed her Tucson Symphony Orchestra season tickets adding, "I might as well be an optimist, pessimism sucks!" I, too, renew season tickets for all the classical music in Tucson. Live music is always the highlight of my day. But I allow myself to give the tickets away if I am too tired to attend a concert.

I try to obey my "Only one thing a day" rule. What is a "thing"? It is an event for which I look in the mirror to make sure I am appropriately dressed and coifed (hair up instead of pony-tailed). It has a time to arrive as for a meeting, a lunch, a concert or movie. It is on my calendar as I no longer trust my brain to remind me of anything.

I have minimized my "things" by resigning from all boards and community obligations. (Disclosure for fact-checkers: I permit my name to be listed on a letterhead as long as I am not expected to attend meetings.) No more dinners with friends before a concert, that's for people newly on Medicare.

Letting it go. This is what I call the Scarlett O'Hara approach to mental health. To quote, "I can't think about that right now. If I do, I'll go crazy. I'll think about that tomorrow." This strategy is especially useful to us oldies. By tomorrow we may have forgotten all about it!

Keeping busy works for me provided I stop before exhaustion sets in. When I was writing my first book, I set an alarm clock for an hour. The alarm reminded me to get up and run around the house a few times to rev up the circulation to my brain and other sit-weary body parts. Can I still run? No way! Just the other day Tucson's sky was filled with glorious clouds making it a perfect day to run for joy. I thought, "Oh, yes, I remember running, it used to be great fun!"

This morning while writing this, I asked my cellphone to alert me in an hour. When the alarm went off I saved my unfinished doc, poured myself a cup of coffee, and (gasp!) finished a novel I was reading. The sky did not fall! I must remember to do this more often! Write that down quick, Marilyn!

I still wrestle with questions like, What is possible and practical for me now? I can't do it all any more, and actually can't do even a portion of what I once did. And the number of such "impossibles" will increase.

This leads to another question, What is really important to me now? For me, and I suspect for most of us, family and friends top the list. I remind myself to focus on what gives me the most pleasure or satisfaction. What I enjoy most is reading and writing ('rithmetic not so much) which fortunately fits with what is still possible.

Earlier in life we were so busy doing what we had to do at work and home we did not have much time to reflect on life. In our later years we have such "reflection" time. I can be more mindful now than when I had two small children and a busy job.

Reflection leads me to the existential questions. How can I accept with grace the reality of my life now? What's next? How do I find equanimity?

For me the answers lie somewhere between realistic acceptance and an optimistic outlook. I have always tried, and still do try, to look for the sunny flip side when the other side is gloomy.

What will happen if I can no longer drive or no longer want to? I will Uber (used it recently when traveling ... easy to do and works great!).

One of the hardest things we elderdrivers face is making the decision to stop driving. Sometimes an accident scares us. Or we start getting tickets that mean our driving is not acceptable to the police. Our spouse or children may notice we should not be driving. Or take the keys away. Safety must supersede our ego. Safety issues are not only about people getting hurt. Being sued for an injury or death due to poor driving that has been documented can also cause harm to our bank account.

By the way, one of the hardest tasks of *my* life was driving my husband to the DMV to replace his driver's license with a card that serves as ID for boarding a plane. I told his doctor that I was worried about his driving and she sent him to evaluate his driving ability. He flunked. He wept leaving the DMV, sobbing that he had been driving since he was 15.

Travel? It is both a challenge and very wonderful. I have had the good fortune to visit 106 countries on this wonderful planet and all 50 states. How come? A love of travel, longevity, and a bit of cheating. I visited the Ukraine when it was part of the USSR. Now it is a separate country so I count it.

Travelling is also arduous, especially at my age. Flying ain't what it used to be when there were no long lines, we had sufficient room for legs and carry-on baggage, and we were fed a meal even in the back of the airplane. My mother wore white gloves because plane travel was considered a special event.

On my first flight in my teens, I was thrilled by the physical act of going up in an airplane. I was moving faster in space than ever before! I always intended to take flying lessons but never did. It is in my still unfilled bucket list along with a few countries I never saw like Cambodia and Vietnam. But my bucket was filled with so many wonderful places I cannot complain. And I have not ruled out travel completely, not yet anyhow.

When traveling becomes too much for me, I will reflect on past travels dusting off the many travel journals and photographs I have kept.

I will continue to appreciate nature though I no longer hike. I feel grateful to be alive on this beautiful planet and will do everything I can to preserve and protect our earth. I can still type my protests even if I no longer march on behalf of the environment. My fingers march to sign checks supporting issues I care about.

I will continue to relish one part of me that is still intact: my curiosity. We are lucky to be alive at a time when it has never been easier to satisfy our curiosity on any subject. Thanks to Google it only takes a few clicks instead of a trip to the library.

I keep myself informed, reading two newspapers every day, a bunch of periodicals, and as many books as possible. Taking courses simply for the fun of learning something new is still a treat.

As we advance in age, we face an uncertain path to an inescapable future. The future has always been uncertain but in youth one rarely thinks about it. Now each of us in our own way must amble along searching like Diogenes to find our own honest truth about the meaning of life.

Facing the truth of our present and past years can lead us to gratitude for what we had, appreciation of what we still have, and strength to face our future. We can renew feelings of optimism as well as symphony tickets. Pessimism sucks!

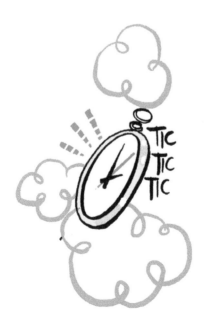

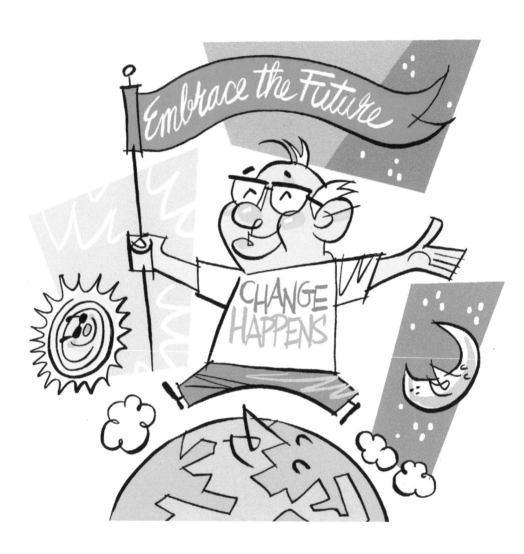

CHAPTER 9

OH, THE CHANGES YOU WILL SEE!

Dr. Seuss is one of my heroes! He wrote marvelous books for children but he also educated parents. He could get to the core of humans and their relationships better than many writers.

The last book he wrote and illustrated was, *Oh, the Places You'll Go!* published in 1990. A reviewer: the book describes the journey of life and its challenges. Me: the book exalts going forth without fear. A great message for children and for us living in Geriatrica as well.

Life is a journey. A journey means changes. A journey means learning about new places.

I am happy that I am still very curious about the world. Curiosity starts at birth when baby seeks and sees mother's face. All our lives we try to make sense of the world and ourselves. I still love to learn new things and make connections to what I already know ... even if I forget some of them!

My own life changed when I moved from the frozen north to Tucson in the summer of 1979 to become an associate dean at the medical school. I had always lived north of the 42nd parallel close to either an ocean or a big lake.

The first thing I had to learn was the meaning of the word "hot." I found out from my blistered fingers what the desert heat does to metal like car door handles and mailboxes. And quickly learned that one does not run to the bank at lunchtime in the summer. Actually, this one didn't run at all. I also learned to walk on the shady side of the street.

My shopping list now includes copious supplies of sunscreen, moisturizer, and eye drops. A water bottle became my constant companion and that's how I learned the location of every accessible restroom in Tucson.

My dog quickly learned the First Commandment for Tucson Canines, "Always Poop in the Shade."

I discovered the blessings of dawn in the desert. And the glorious dusks! Bliss to sit outdoors with a cool drink watching the beautiful sunsets. And later seeing the stars pop out one by one in the darkening sky.

I quickly came to love my new job and hometown. I remember my first trip to the then bustling El Con Mall. People around me were chattering in Spanish. Neat! I could hear an exotic language without flying to another country! Though adjusting to the desert itself took a while, now I cannot imagine living anywhere else!

Those of us now in Geriatrica have lived through lots of events as our world spun. I was born in 1930 so I can remember the Great Depression. Even I could tell it was a time of scarcity. I saw hungry people begging for food on street corners and at our back door. My father lost his job and the job he was lucky to get paid a lot less. I never knew hunger myself but could imagine it and the shame of begging.

I lived through WW II, the Korean War, Vietnam, the Cold War, etc. Newsreels scared me and made me feel grateful I was not being bombed. And turned me into a lifelong pacifist. I fantasized about the UN creating an International Guard. Young men from all over the world would train together every summer and stop every conflict between nations quickly. The soldiers would get to know and like each other so much that no wars would ever start! The silly notion of a young girl but I still think it might work!

My generation saw and experienced a multitude of changes. My family bought a secondhand car! Street cars disappeared.

Interstate highways crisscrossed our beautiful country and made it possible for us to drive over hills and dales to Grandmother's house. But trains dwindled, and were replaced by gas-guzzling cars that did not help us lower our carbon footprint.

Levittown started the single home craze for nearly all families. The corner drugstore and family-owned grocery store morphed into brightly-lit supermarkets. Malls appeared to take the place of the neighborhood clothing establishment and department stores. Fast food restaurants! Movies in color! Multiplex movie theatres! Ice boxes became refrigerators that made ice! Air-conditioning!

Phones changed from the party line to the black dial model that sat on a square telephone table, to colored phones everywhere, and then to cellphones glued to everyone's ear.

In the 40s my father, an electrical engineer, was given a TV set by the embryonic Boston TV station before it began to broadcast. He would be alerted by telephone when the TV station sent out a test pattern to see if it worked. When TV broadcasting started, we had the first TV on the block! Neighbors were invited, still more neighbors asked to come see this new wonder. Our parlor was always filled. I don't remember what we watched in black and white. But I do remember what my mother said when the sofa broke and had to be replaced. "TV causes sofas to break!"

Cable invaded our homes giving us a bushel of channels. That is changing now. I am just beginning a relationship with Alexa ... but there is a learning curve. However, when the blue light at the top of the Fire Cube lights up and Alexa finds me my wanted movie in a nanosecond, I love her!

The Internet has changed us tremendously. This is both a blessing and a curse. Social media has invaded our lives with blessings like FaceTime for grandparents and curses for society because it can spread hate so rapidly and destructively.

Changes in medicine, public health, and science have been stupendous! Death rates from infectious diseases and heart disease have plummeted. If it weren't for the (I can't print the adjective) opioid epidemic, the availability of guns, increasing suicide rates, obesity driven by corn farmers who gave us high-fructose corn syrup, and health care for only some, our national statistics would be even better. We the people would be healthier!

All of us Geriatricians have witnessed tremendous changes in our life and world, especially in medicine and technology. Never have the "changes you'll see" happened so fast! And no day will go by without us hearing of another amazing new technological change. Can we foresee or predict?

Thomas Friedman of *The New York Times* writes that the old binary left/right way of thinking about issues and world problems isn't going to work now. Things are accelerating too fast. He quotes Linton Wells, " ... to find the solutions to today's wicked problems you should never think in the box and never think out of the box. You have to think without a box."

Heather McGowan, future-of-work strategist, says things we have to make decisions about are so interdependent, "... our old two-dimensional grid with its binary choices ... requires a more complex, three-dimensional set of policy tools and responses."

The way I look at things today, if we have the new tasks of adjusting quickly plus having to think in a whole new way, we certainly need the perspectives of both Age and Youth. We need grandparents and grandkids to keep talking to each other and learning from each other. There is enough division in our crazy world!

The extended family may be scattered to the four corners of the world but grandparents can and should try to teach the grandchildren about their world and the children should teach us about theirs. (See Chapter 22.)

Grandparents, stay connected to your grandchildren in all ways possible. In person whenever possible, but when you are separated by geography, give thanks for the technology we already have. The telephone, texting, Facebook, and FaceTime are all a gift to grandparents.

I get occasional questions from grandparents who are not technically savvy. My advice to them: Develop a relationship with a computer ASAP. Don't let technology scare you. Even though your computer can do everything but bake banana bread, start out with just the basics especially email and Googling.

I know next to nothing about the inner workings of my computer or how many things it can do with a better-informed owner, but we have a pretty good relationship nonetheless.

I have learned that computers, like people, get cranky sometimes and do not behave as expected. Learn to SAVE your work frequently and perform a RESTART to help the crankiness. It's like when you get up and make yourself a cup of tea.

One writer friend says she knows how very little about her beloved computer that helps her make a living. "But what I can do, I do very well!" I have a computer guru who helps me out by phone when a restart does not work. Everybody knows computers do these things only when there is a looming deadline.

I learned to text when I realized it was the best way to reach grandkids these days. My clumsy fingertips can type out a short message like "Call me." or "Check the email I just sent." But typing is lots easier on a real keyboard. And reading on a big screen is easier than reading on a smart phone.

I call to ask my grandchildren about their school or job but I also ask for their take on the world today. There are rapid cultural changes I want to know more about. I ask a lot of: "What does it feel like to ... ?" and "Do many of your generations feel the way you do about ... ?"

It is fascinating to cross the generations gap. I learn much about these people I love and about the Land of Youth they live in. As I don't query any adults about their love life or criticize what they are wearing, I don't do these things to my grown grandchildren either.

The relationship between grandparents and grandchildren is vitally important to both. It is not a one-way street, we learn from each other. Remember "Don't ask, don't tell?" Grandparents should both ask and tell, but in the reverse order. Tell your grandchildren about your life, your victories and your defeats, even your mistakes. When an older person shares, younger ones get the message that it's OK for them to share.

Some families find it easier to talk than others do. They see each other as often as possible but spend the time feasting and catching up on what everybody is doing. Not how they are feeling. A bold grandparent could share feelings about aging to start a deeper conversation ball rolling.

Grandparents are able to transcend daily parenting interactions so they have time to share facts, feelings, and memories. Let's use this ability to teach our grandchildren about aging and to learn about youth today.

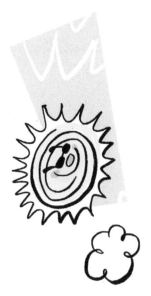

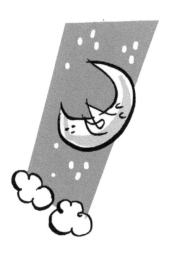

YOUR MAP

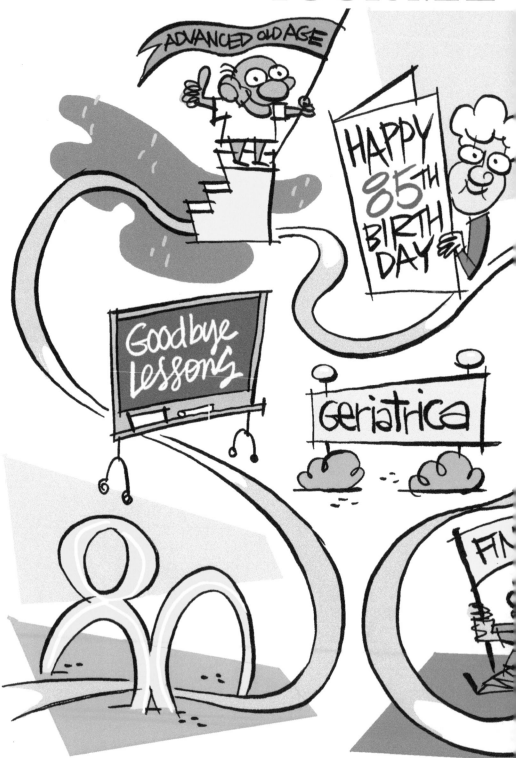

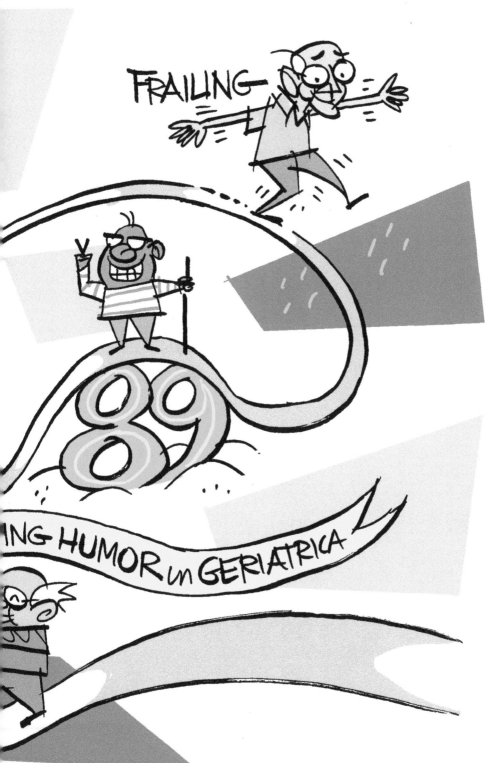

FRAILING

89

ING HUMOR in GERIATRICA

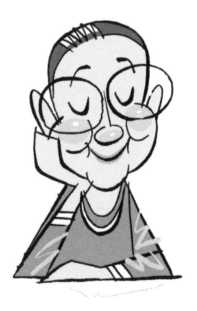

PART II INTRODUCTION

MY PERSONAL ODYSSEY

In looking back, my immigration journey to Geriatrica started in earnest when I reached 80 years of age.

Aging starts at birth and is official when we reach 65. That was the traditional get-your-gold-watch retirement age. Happy Mom and Pop, released from the daily grind, bought an RV and traveled all over. At Yellowstone Park about 20 years ago I overheard a young park worker tell his buddy, "Here come the raisins!" waiting for a bus load of elderly people to slowly disembark. We had a grandchild with us so when we boarded the bus I muttered, "Here come two raisins and one grape!"

Part II is more or less a diary of my personal observations over a decade. Unlike a traditional daily diary, I wrote these a year or so apart. They touch on how I felt each year. Tempus fugit ... and so do our thoughts!

Immigrating to Geriatrica, or anywhere, is a journey. The housewives, immigrating in a covered wagon to homestead the vast American West, often kept a diary. I suggest my fellow elders mark each birthday by jotting down a few words about your own journey, what you did and how you felt.

Happy aging!

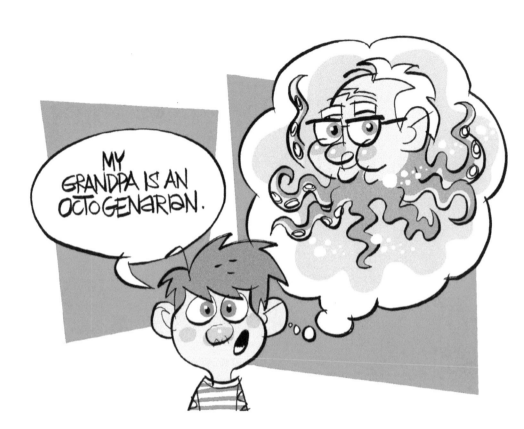

CHAPTER 10

BECOMING AN OCTOGENARIAN

Wow! I have lived long enough to call myself an octogenarian.

I joined a pretty select group of people on my 80th birthday. I wonder about my fellow oldies. How are other people 80 and above faring?

I shared some data in Chapter 1, but curiosity urged me on. The median age for women in the United States is 39.4; for men, 36.8. I am above average, in age anyway!

Women live longer than men do. We are more prone to depression. But we are more social. So if we outlive our spouse we do better living alone than men do.

Limitations? Yes, 55 percent of all people over 80 reported a severe disability and 29 percent of these required assistance.

Chronic conditions? People are living longer with chronic conditions. There has been a 50 percent decrease in death rates for heart disease and stroke thanks to better treatment. Thus, as many as 90 percent of us have one or more chronic conditions including me and just about everyone I know. Diabetes in the elderly is increasing due to obesity.

Most paid and unpaid caregivers are women. Yes, they are not paid enough. Women often have to leave work to care for an ailing spouse and this reduces household income and leaves many in financial hardship when the spouse dies.

Nearly one third of older adults not living in a facility are alone. Being alone is not healthy especially as we get even older and leave the house less often.

As we age the years seem to fly past at supersonic speed. My own unscientific Theory of Relativity is that time moves slowly when we are young. Remember how long it took for the minute hand to creep from 2:59 to 3:00 when you were in first grade? Now the years go by so fast my head spins.

We actually start aging when we are born. Let me correct myself, we start aging when we are in the womb.

A Cambridge University study showed that rats submitted to less oxygen in the womb were born with shortened telomeres due to the stress. Telomeres are like caps on the ends of our DNA strands protecting them. Each time one of our cells divides the telomeres get shorter until they get so short the cell cannot divide anymore and it becomes inactive or dies. Telomere shortening is a scientific marker associated with aging.

A simpler way of saying this is that life has a mortality rate of 100 percent. No one gets out of life alive. Time goes in only one direction. We will never again be a newborn!

Many of us begin to feel tiny hints of aging at about age 40. We notice we just aren't like we were at 35 anymore! Glasses are needed about age 45 when presbyopia (this means old eyes) appears. Some hints of chronic disease appears like hypertension. Menopause occurs about age 50.

Personally, I felt great at 50. My children were launched. My career and marriage were humming along nicely. At about age 65 I could no longer ignore that I was slowing down. Some creaky joints start to ache, stronger glasses needed, my hearing was going, a couple of chronic problems crept in.

But I still hiked and camped in our creaky, cramped but reliable cabover camper. I traveled the world, was active in medical education and the women's movement on a national level, and served on community boards.

I never imagined that there would be so many new things to learn in my senior years. I must learn how to deal with a rapidly changing world and my aging body. I struggle to accept my diminishing energy, speed, stamina, and strength. The rhythm of my life has changed because everything takes longer to do.

But when I think of the alternative, I feel blessed! Life is a gift for us and for those people who love us. Whatever comes don't look a gift horse in the mouth! This translates into don't question the value of a gift. Always wondered where this saying came from so I looked it up. Horse traders learned the age and worth of a horse by looking at its teeth.

The best way of putting age in perspective is to attend as many 100th-year birthday parties as possible (including our own!). Inspiring events! Speeches from many including the birthday person. People think about how much the honoree has seen.

This gives us a jump start on thinking about all we have seen in our own life on earth.

I am grateful for and remember all the beautiful places I have been privileged to see. I have watched my family grow and prosper. We octogenarians have seen enormous strides in medicine that enabled many of us to still be here. I witnessed some amazing things to help people like the Marshall Plan and the GI Bill.

"What a ride we have had, Sam! What glorious Ups and devastating Downs," I told the new centenarian.

My ride started in the Great Depression. My father lost his job and my parents had to move in with my mother's family. My parents looked at the bright side, "Things can't get any worse, let's have a baby!" That baby was me.

I remember the Depression, World War II, the Cold War, Korea, Vietnam, Iraq, Afghanistan, 9/11. We have seen much political turmoil and upheaval, enormous strides in medicine coupled with egregious lack of coverage for many, decline in our once glorious public education system, significant negative changes in the family, outrageous refusal to face the impact of our energy consumption on the planet, our polarized, dysfunctional government, burgeoning inequality, and the corporate takeover of America. We have become a nation of the corporations, by the corporations, and for the corporations that all have lobbyists. The customer is always right, right? Naah ... people no longer count except as consumers who increase profits for the stockholders and the wealth of those at the top.

What keeps me sane? What keeps all of us sane in a world of 24-hour news? I turn off the TV when Breaking News becomes No Longer News. More important, I reflect on the 60s, that transformative decade. On January 1, 1960, I never even dreamed that in the next 10 years I would witness the passage of Civil Rights legislation, the doubling of the number of women accepted to law and medical school, and most important the start of the slow but continuing change in how people feel toward those different from themselves. Only we are far from Utopia (and the 60s was a decade with many horrific events as well as social progress) but many Americans changed their ways of thinking about these things. Who knows, maybe another transformative decade is around the corner.

As I aged I have learned to worship that glorious product of evolution: the human brain. The most complicated entity in the universe. Wouldn't it be wonderful if we could use our brains to arrive at beautiful solutions not horrible, hurtful things. If we could stop making decisions based on our differences, but on the inescapable fact that we are one people on a fragile planet and need to work together.

I hope we choose the right path, before we end up with no choice at all like Woody Allen. In a *New Yorker* piece about giving a commencement address he wrote, "More than at any other time in history, mankind faces a crossroads. One path leads to despair and utter hopelessness. The other, to total extinction. Let us pray we have the wisdom to choose correctly."

Yes, let all of us strive toward beautiful solutions for all peoples while we still can.

What is my advice for those of us who have been around a while? I plan to think about the momentous events I lived through. When memory fails I Google: "events in 19__" to glance through what happened that year.

Look back on your own life span, reflect on the progress and problems you have seen. Write it all down and also talk to your children and grandchildren. Remind them that they are the ones who can make the beautiful solutions happen.

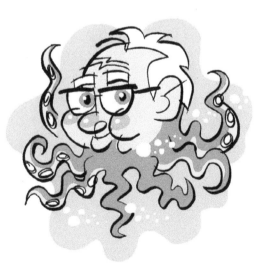

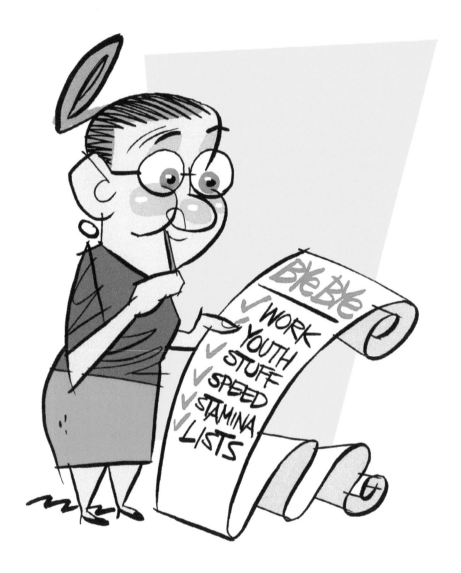

CHAPTER 11

GOODBYE LESSONS

I accepted the fact that I was aging. But it was not until my 80s that I realized I was GETTING OLD! My strength, speed and stamina continued to decrease. Everything was slowing down.

I have had to make some baby step changes. The morning walk diminished from four miles to two. Hiking on uneven paths was over. I stopped cooking big festive meals for holidays. A friend said she could still cook up a storm but always had to spend the next two days in bed!

I made a vow that I would never, ever step on a ladder or a stepstool again. Safety first. I was alone one night at about 10 pm when my smoke detector started screaming at me. I tried to reach the damn thing but even on tiptoes, my fingertips were an arms length away from it. Fortunately, the lights were still on in a neighbor's house. He did not even need a stepstool! What seemed like ten seconds later the screaming stopped and a new battery was installed. I love my neighbors!

I must confess that aging astonishes me! I never imagined that there would be so many new things to learn in my senior years. I must learn how to deal with a rapidly changing world, loss of loved ones, and my aging body. I struggle to accept my diminishing energy, speed, and stamina. The rhythm of my life has changed because everything takes longer to do.

Longevity is a special blessing for those with good enough health and the means to live independently. We oldies know the math and understand that most of our lifetimes have already been lived. But, as a wise woman told me after my husband's death, "There is a new chapter in your life yet to be written." This is a good perspective from which to view what is ahead.

Adjusting to aging means adjusting to change, a no-brainer. But how? After much soul searching I have come to believe the process starts with saying "Goodbye!" as cheerfully as possible, to what was and saying "Hello!" to what will come.

This is a lot easier said than done. My mother, who died at age 99, lived alone in a house that had become too much for her, surrounded by a garden she could no longer walk in, let alone care for, and that sad kind of loneliness that results from outliving practically everybody. She refused to move. Mom, how about an apartment near where one of us lives? A senior facility? Her answer never varied. "I will not leave my house, I don't want to change a thing in my house, I don't even want to talk about it."

Why this strong resistance to change as we age? Is it an exaggeration of how some of us were always reluctant to change? Is it a phenomenon of aging? Are we unwilling to make changes because we like our old surroundings so well? Do we fear the unfamiliar? Is it that we don't have the energy to change?

Probably all of the above. But I suspect reluctance to change may also be related to the fact we are so acquisitive. Our culture teaches us from early childhood to acquire and value our acquisitions. The message: Get a college education, an advanced degree, a spouse, children, a house, a bigger house, furnishings, and other worldly goods, cars, flat abs and hard biceps at the gym, souvenirs from our travels. Acquire! Acquire more!

But nobody teaches us to say goodbye. Grief counselors help us deal with enforced goodbyes—a death, a debilitating illness. But what about learning how to voluntarily say goodbye to an old way of life, to possessions that are becoming too much for us, to our old methods of doing things and thinking about the world?

Perhaps we seniors need goodbye lessons. If we learn to say goodbye, maybe we will have more space within our core selves to say hello to something new. But if we don't learn to push the "delete" button on at least some of the old things, there's no room for anything new. Change doesn't have a chance. How about Goodbye Classes and Goodbye Group Therapy for seniors to help those who can't get started in the process of letting go?

I sense danger for myself in refusing to change as my mother did. All we can expect in our world as we age is change, likely to be more radical than ever before because of technology. All we can expect from ourselves is that we will become less able to do things we could once do.

To help me accept the inevitable changes to come, I have started taking some goodbye baby steps. Life has been good to me. I have not had to deal with too many "emergency" goodbyes like deaths or disabilities. But I have started some "elective" goodbyes.

My first step was to become deliberately less acquisitive. I have enough "stuff" and I don't need anything else to shop for, unwrap, put away, and worry about. (Disclaimer: Books and CDs are not considered stuff in this house so they continue to overflow my shelves.) However, I did learn it is possible to travel overseas, even to an exotic destination, and not bring back anything except memories and a few photographs.

Acquiring things takes time. Learning the art of **not** acquiring gives us more time, now our most precious commodity. Plus, we don't have to dig into tightly sealed cartons or struggle with shrink wrap (a special hell for aging fingers). If we accept the premise you can't take it with you, why not decrease the burden of watching and fussing over "it" before we actually go.

I am also beginning to divest myself of possessions. My children are getting keepsakes and other items "early" while local charities benefit from that which we all accumulate but don't need.

I gradually relinquish some work hours replacing them with time for contemplation and enjoying, instead of regretting, the slower pace at which I live. The slower pace brings a special joy and awe that comes from recognizing how beautiful the world is and what a privilege it is to be alive.

Worries persist. A friend said recently, "Everybody I know is gone or going." All seniors fear losing their independence, a realistic worry. Based on what my mother did not do, I am looking at senior facilities now in order to prepare for a day when I may no longer be able to live independently. To my way of thinking having such concerns is the price we pay for longevity ... a fair price all things considered.

Perhaps the acts of saying goodbye we learn will one day be hailed as a healthy practice for senior citizens. MRIs could even demonstrate that aging brains light up in living color, revealing the new connections we make when saying goodbye to the old and hello to the new.

Let's all try it!

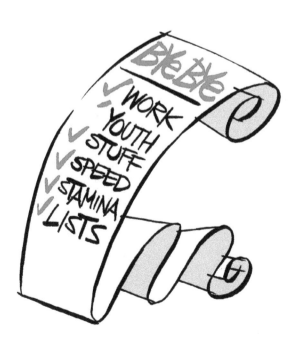

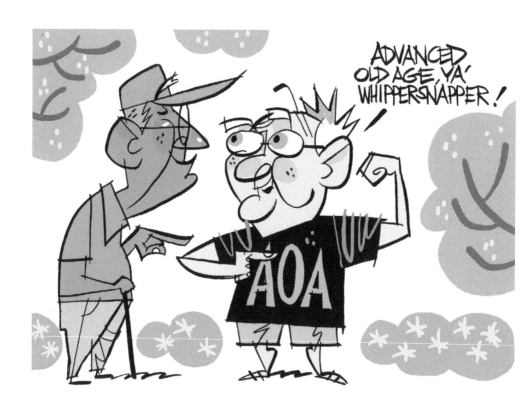

CHAPTER 12

ADVANCED OLD AGE

I can say with certitude that I have now entered Advanced Old Age (AOA). What is it and how do I know I'm there? I note little losses everywhere, except of course, in ever-persistent belly fat.

We each enter AOA at different times depending on our health, our genes, the circumstances of our lives, and our outlook on life. Some bodily changes like sagging flesh are not a major problem, but illness or a fall that puts you in a wheelchair can speed up the process.

Myself? I notice slower walking, more difficulty in retrieving memories, slower thinking, less energy, even a tad less enthusiasm to do things I like to do. I call this the stay-home-and-stream instead of go-out-tonight phenomenon.

Pediatricians work with adolescents as well as babies. It never occurred to me until quite recently the many similarities between AOA and adolescence. Both going through adolescence and advancing into old age brings a multitude of changes.

Puberty brings changes to just about every part of the body. There are changes in size, shape, sex organs, skin, senses. Teens feel funny in this new body and worry what others think. Their brain is beginning to develop new connections especially in the prefrontal area where reasoning, planning, judgment and other grownup kinds of thinking reside. And mood changes occur with lightning speed.

AOA can bring many bodily changes. We sag, stoop, shrink,

see and hear less well. Our cognitive changes are opposite those in a teenager. We both lose connections in our aging brain and greatly increase our retrieval time. You know this is happening to you when you remember the name of the person you talked to at the party, but two days later. On the positive side we don't get zits.

Other positives: None of us care whether we are pretty or handsome enough to be popular. We are too busy worrying where we put the car keys. Both teens and our group worry those statisticians who keep track of auto accident rates. If there were a contest both have higher than average auto accidents. The teens drive pretty well but are risk-takers. We oldies make up for the fact we have diminished vision, hearing, and neck flexibility to see who's coming up on the right by having a lifetime of driving experience and judgment that teens lack.

The biggest difference is, of course, we have less time ahead. We are winding down not gearing up. By the time we qualify for AOA most of us have come to grips with our numbered days. Our teenage grandchildren may wonder how it feels to be in the last years of life. Can there be a plus?

If anyone asks me this question my answer is a loud yes! We feel lucky to still be around, to have escaped all the illnesses and accidents that could have befallen us. I think our bodies are telling us something: slow down so we have more time to appreciate what we have.

Do I have any advice for those who approach AOA? Remember, until very recently I spent more time writing about adolescents and babies than the elderly. But this is what I have learned from my personal odyssey.

Focus on and be grateful on what is left, not what is gone. Keep as active as you can. Do not shut yourself up in AOA ... stay connected in person, phone, video chats.

An adolescent slams the door of his or her room to mope or sulk. If you feel mopey, OK mope but set a timer. Allow yourself 20 minutes for the pity party, then eat a square of chocolate saved for these moments, and soldier on. Why 20 minutes? Think of it this way, unlike the teen, we don't have a lifetime ahead of us so let's not waste what time we have moping.

Stay curious. Take courses, keep informed and keep reading ... it's good for the brain. Go outdoors. Try to see a sunrise and a sunset and stars every day. That means three times outdoors ... good for the soul. Spend some time with younger folks. Don't try to be who you are not. Rock concert attendance is not necessary and could kill off the rest of your hearing, but I always feel refreshed after being with children or young people. Keep moving as best you can. Can't work out at the gym any longer? Walk, with a cane if necessary. Accept help with gratitude. Offer help to others when you can. Don't fall!

Bottom line for me: I would not want to be an adolescent again. I'd have to make all those big life decisions and go through all those life changes. Perhaps the best comparison between teens and oldies is that we are now our own boss. I can make my own decisions and, if the time comes that I cannot, I have left specific directives and have confidence in those who will make decisions for me.

My mother who died at age 99 used to say, "I'm out of it!" when people were discussing things like politics. I thought that was a wrong attitude, however now I suspect she was happy not to bother about such things. I am far from "out of it" today but if the time comes when I feel I am ready to let others solve the world's problems, that's OK too ... as long as I can still read good literature and listen to beautiful music.

Speaking of beautiful music, recently I began hearing music in my head. Sometimes I wake up to it or it comes to my consciousness whenever it pleases. Sometimes I realize why a certain melody comes to me as I can trace the connections. Other times I have no idea why Beethoven's "Ode to Joy" pops into my head.

Sometimes the music becomes an "ear worm" playing over and over again. As our ears don't store anything except wax, I prefer to call this a brain worm. I am thrilled I have all this beautiful music in my brain so I don't have to get up and take a CD out of its sleeve.

Just to be sure I asked my psychiatrist daughter about this phenomenon. She told me I am not hearing things, as in hallucinations. "Don't worry, Mom, enjoy the concerts!"

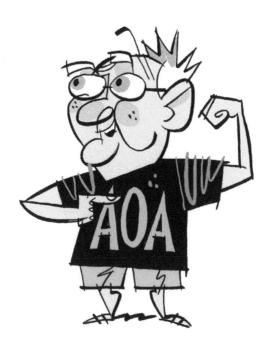

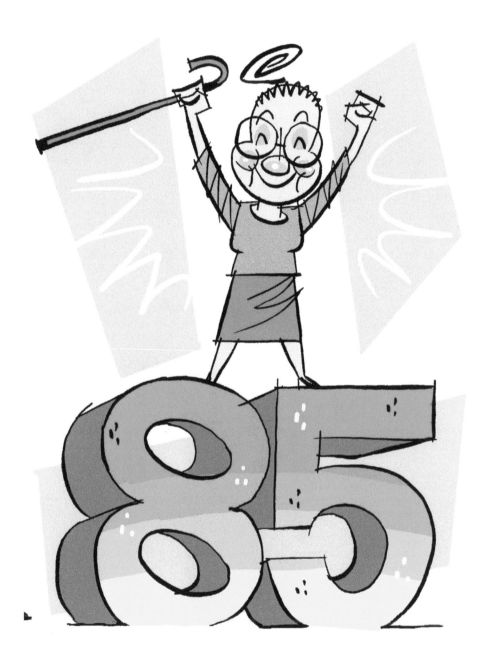

CHAPTER 13

REACHING 85

It's official. I am now a little old lady ... LOL. Reaching 85 is a milestone alright. But the magnitude of the number 85 gives one pause! It takes a long time to count slowly from one to 85.

I am not at all bothered by unimportant stuff like looks. I ignore my sagging belly and neck, as well as the fact that my wrinkles have developed wrinkles of their own. No one can break the law of gravity. How we look in our later years is a sort of tax we pay for the privilege of longevity on this beautiful planet.

I admit I am bothered by how my aging body functions. I am grateful that I can still walk and talk and drive. But I get terribly cross with my aging fingers. It seems to take me longer to open a package than the time it took for the Amazon Prime delivery to reach my front door. We need a scissors in every room, pliers must always be handy to open a bottle of bubbly or even a stubborn bottle of water. Don't even mention the words "shrink wrap" or I get hysterical.

I remember learning in medical school that aging skin loses both elasticity and subcutaneous tissue thereby becoming fragile. But who knew that the mere touch of a featherweight object against one's arm could cause bruising, or that bruises get bruised if brushed again?

Old ladies have to balance and walk carefully. A carefree walk down a flight of stairs without clutching the handrail is a thing of the past. Donning trifocals and hearing aids becomes a part of one's daily dressing routine. Calendar meltdown occurs if I don't immediately write down something I have to remember like who, when, and where I just arranged to meet for lunch. And woe will be to the aged person who lets more than a nanosecond pass before adding toilet paper to the shopping list.

Because many of us begin to run out of strength, speed, and stamina even before we get our Medicare card, oldies can only avoid near-terminal fatigue by careful planning. Though I could once handle three "things" a day (taking a class, dinner out, and a concert) I cannot do it now. As a matter of fact, cooking dinner before an evening event can be too taxing. This is why I invented the avocado sandwich requiring only two ingredients, one plate, no cooking.

Remember how important perfection once was? For me it was a joy to accomplish a task quickly and perfectly. I didn't need or expect praise. I needed my own pat on the back: a silent, "Great job, Marilyn!"

These days I am learning how to settle for less than perfect. Opera lovers will chuckle over my gradual acceptance of the "Boris" concept. One family I know used the term to describe a task that was done good enough. As in *Boris Godunov.* I can now tolerate a less than perfectly made bed or dusted table. Warning: The Boris concept is not to be used in matters of health or safety!

Time is now precious. It always has been but when we are young we don't realize it. I am increasingly bothered by things that waste my time. Like unwanted phone calls or the eternity it takes to reach a real person when what you need is not available on any button you are told to press.

Like many other octogenarians, I am an immigrant in a digital world and speak the language haltingly. I am hopelessly CSL (Computer as Second Language). The many things my smarter-than-I-am gadgets can do bewilder me. And a 12-year-old grandchild is not always at hand.

Because the Land of Geriatrica is a new territory for me, life feels strange sometimes. Most of us are retired and have been out of school for many years. Yet we must continue to learn new things about a rapidly changing world and our own changing capabilities. I actually spend more time these days giving advice to myself than I do to parents. Sometimes the advice is pretty similar.

Many years ago, I wrote that every child needs the three essential Parenting Vitamin A's: affection, attention, and acceptance. Now I realize we oldies need to parent ourselves the same way. Be **affectionate** to yourself. Cut yourself some slack. Learn to comfort yourself like a parent would.

Pay **attention** to yourself. Tend to your needs. Reward yourself with a treat for accomplishing a task even if it took you longer than it did when you were young and feisty.

Most important, **accept** yourself for who you are now. You will never be the young person you once were. But you're still here so be a good parent to yourself ... and to any other old people in your life.

More essentials to ponder: the need for connections, curiosity, and compassion. As we age, we need **connections** to others. We must guard against isolation and loneliness. We should start thinking about ways to be with others long before the time comes when we can no longer drive or manage a house.

Curiosity about the world keeps my mind active. I Google new things (or, these days, things I have forgotten) many times a day taking advantage of one of the digital world's blessings. Much easier than going to a library, holding a heavy dictionary, or bending down to get a volume of the encyclopedia.

We may be old but we are human beings so we must continue, as long as we are able, to offer **compassion** to others. And, when the time comes, gracefully and gratefully accept the compassion of others.

Aging, if we are lucky, can be much more than pesky losses. There is richness in our many years of memories. Recalling a lifetime of people and places. Hearing a melody and remembering when you first heard it as a child. Rereading a great book like *Anna Karenina* and thinking what a different person you were when you read it as an adolescent.

Every day can bring simple pleasures. The joys of seeing family and friends. Walking the dog in the early morning. Watching the sunset. An email from a dear friend who is far away. A phone call from a three-year-old grandchild.

Make peace with any regrets, we cannot change the past. Enjoy all your happy memories. The great American philosopher, Dr.

Seuss, wrote, "Don't cry because it's over, smile because it happened."

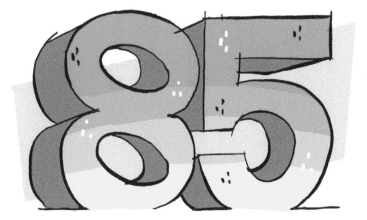

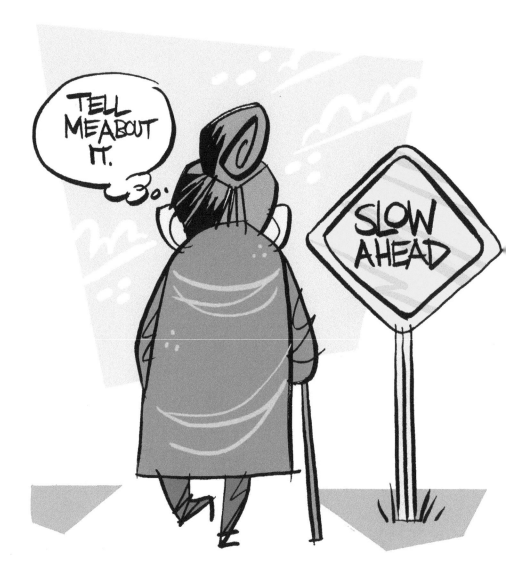

CHAPTER 14

FRAILING

My 88th birthday! A humongous number no matter which way you look at it. Fellow-travelers who are in advanced old age may chuckle when I write I am an Old(s) 88. My musician son just told me I have lived a year for every key on the piano keyboard!

How am I doing? I used to answer that I was still vertical, but I hereby coin a new word. When people ask me how I am, my answer is I am "frailing." It means I am not quite yet frail but I can see fragility on the horizon ... with my good glasses of course.

Frail is a word I would never have used to describe myself until recently. Chunky, maybe. Robust. Energetic. Hard-working. But I am definitely slowing down.

I walk slower and very carefully. My creaky knee troubles me. Balance is something I have to think about ... a far cry from that little girl on a bike or the woman on a tough hiking trail that once I was. Plumbing problems plague me so a restroom is the first thing I look for wherever I go. There are several prescription drugs to keep track of. I forget more easily and recall less speedily.

On the positive side, I am doing pretty good when I compare myself to others my age. I am still alive while, of every 100,000 white females born the year I was born, only 37, 745 are still alive. Life expectancy for females at age 88 is 5.6 years. Males do not fare quite as well: for every 100,000 white males born in 1930 only 25,139 are living and life expectancy is 4.4 years.

These are statistical analyses, not guarantees. When we are young we know our life will end but don't pay much attention to the passing of time. Maybe because life is so fulfilling and interesting the future seems endless. But now even those of us who weren't good at math can count the possible number of days we may have left.

The epitaph of the book *Number Our Days* by Barbara Myerhoff about elderly Jews is a prayer adapted from two psalms that ends "So teach us to number our days, that we may get us a heart of wisdom." We oldies know our days are numbered. Let us hope we also get us a heart of wisdom so that we can accept ourselves as we are today. And that our wisdom helps us do our damnedest to enjoy each day.

We all need to pay attention to two things that can affect both the quality and length of our lives. Our wise parents had us immunized against deadly childhood diseases. Now we have to "immunize" ourselves against loneliness and falls, two important risk factors for both mortality and morbidity like a disability.

The immunization is a process of accepting who we are now and what our capabilities are. And accepting the fact that, like time, the trajectory of our "frailing" goes in only one direction. There is no Fountain of Youth.

LONELINESS

"Loneliness as a Public Health Issue" published in *The American Journal of Public Health* is a study of people 60 and over. Those who reported chronic loneliness visited a physician significantly more times than those who were not lonely. Loneliness is a health risk associated with hypertension, risky behaviors like inactivity and smoking, and dementia.

The "Grey Gender Gap" described by Paula Span in *The New York Times* noted that elderly males are more likely to be married than females. Women live longer and generally marry men who are older. Thus women are more likely than men to be widowed and live alone. And, sadly, a higher percentage of elderly women live in poverty. However elderly men living alone do not fare as well as women who are more connected with friends and relatives. Widowers no longer have a wife to supervise their social life and health care.

Is there a cure for loneliness? Yes, friends and activity. The positive effects of people in the lives of the elderly are well known, especially people who live alone.

My husband died when I was 87. In order to survive my grief, I kept busy with activities, concerts, movies, classes ... anything that got me out of the of the house. Mornings were tough. But my beloved Mindy got me up for our walk together. If I had nothing planned that day, I would go to the local coffee house so that I could see and hear people.

I realized there were two aspects to living alone. One was loneliness. My many friends helped me deal with that. But I also experienced "aloneness." Coming home to an empty house with no one to talk to about it made the joys less joyful and the woes more woeful.

Aging makes us less able to avoid both loneliness and aloneness. This is why I am planning to move to an independent living facility (See Chapter 5) where I will have both people and activities on site.

FALLS

Falls can be devastating and life-altering. Nothing can turn us frail more quickly. In old age we have slower reflexes, less coordination and muscle strength, loss of proprioception (the ability to know where our body is in space), and visual problems.

Look around your home with a critical eye and eliminate "fall traps" like scatter rugs or room rugs that are curling up at the edges. Do away with or safely store boxes of "Stuff I am going to go through any day now." Make sure lighting is adequate for your aging eyes. Use night lights for the inevitable trip to the bathroom. Install grab bars in the shower and tub. Ditto rails on steps. Use rails in public buildings and walk slower than usual in new places or in the dark.

Don't ever walk in flimsy shoes or just socks. Use only sensible footwear with corrugated rubber soles. High heels are for models not oldies. Take walks, the best exercise for the elderly. Use a cane if necessary.

Sadly, not all falls can be prevented which means we must do all we can to eliminate the preventable ones. Ironically, while researching and writing this book I had a fall. I wore proper shoes, it was broad daylight but down I went. Nothing broken, a bit of facial blood, a few bruises (my kneecaps are still purple) but I am fully ambulatory. Thankfully I dodged a fall-bullet.

But I have developed PFSD, Post Fall Stress Disorder. I am so scared of another fall I will redouble my efforts to prevent one. Because of travel, family illness, and the death of our dog, I had not been walking and exercising. Back to our morning walk and working with a trainer to strengthen my leg muscles and do special exercises to maintain and improve my balance.

I jokingly asked my trainer if she knew of anyone doing proprioceptor transplants as mine were all gone, my body was bruised from all the things I bump into, and my bruises themselves were getting bruised. Her suggestion was to walk barefoot at home.

I then asked a friend, well-versed in everything neuroscientific, about balance. It's complicated, so complicated I now think of it as a sixth "sense," especially important for the elderly.

Balance depends on our visual system, vestibular system (inner ears and cerebellum), proprioception, and the somatosensory (touch) system. All working together!

Alas, transplanting proprioceptors to our feet won't do it. Walking barefoot does give us information, both proprioceptive and somatosensory, that helps our muscles better respond to what we are walking on and better integrate all the systems that help us balance ourselves.

Challenging our body by doing balance exercises and challenging our feet by walking barefoot can help. Do not do this outside, especially in Arizona, or in unfamiliar places except for a sandy beach.

To keep from becoming frail, I am redoubling my efforts to stay positive in my thinking. I am now working on another kind of balance in my life. I resolve to keep busy but pay attention to when I need a break. And enjoy the quietude of doing absolutely nothing, a new skill for this old lady.

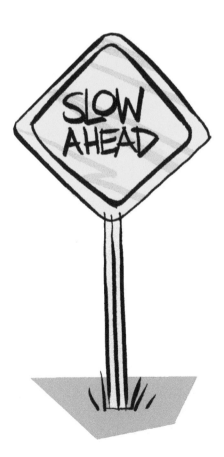

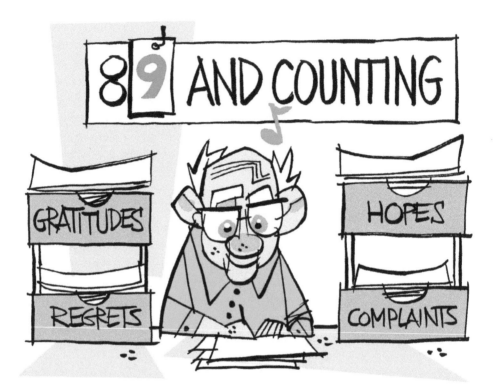

CHAPTER 15

REACHING 89

My 89th birthday! Yes, it's a big number. Next year's birthday will be a monumental one. In case I reach it I better learn, and remember, how to spell nonagenarian!

I am grateful to have reached this milestone. I am privileged to have lived a whole lot of life and accept the reality that I am now squarely in the stage of advanced old age. A white female born in 1930 had a life expectancy of 63.5 years, so I am ahead in the game of longevity. A white female born on the actual date of my birth can expect to live another 5.4 years.

But of course, one's reality is not the same as a cohort bunched together for statistical purposes. An individual is only that, an individual. But numbers do funny things sometimes with no rhyme or reason ... we call it a coincidence. When I was assigned a cell phone number many years ago, it was the year of my birth. I bet not too many people living in Geriatrica can say that!

As I have written before, only the composer gets to write his or her own finale. And it's a totally different kind of finale.

Of course, I have a bunch of complaints but, as of today, I am still vertical and mobile. I have at this writing a stable of medical professionals ... an internist, cardiologist, ophthalmologist, dermatologist, audiologist, and dentist. As I age the list may lengthen.

I am very grateful to be on Medicare. I started paying into Social Security in 1946 when I got my first summer job. I do pay for supplemental insurance and some prescription drugs but shudder to think of what my life and finances would be without Medicare. I shudder even more when I think of people without any health insurance.

I walk nearly every morning. However, I cover way less than the four miles of road I could do before breakfast when I moved here 40 years ago. Now we are the oldest, slowest walkers in the neighborhood. Everybody needs something to brag about, right?

Working out at the gym three times a week is a thing of the past. I still do floor and balance exercises in my home nearly every day but not at the speed or number of reps I once could do. A personal trainer checks in on me to make sure I am doing exercises correctly. Keeping mobile is an important goal for me, as it should be for my readers, so I plan to keep doing these exercises as long as I can still get up from the floor!

Aches and pains persist as I age. To be truthful, they increase but I don't want this chapter to be a downer. A dear friend of my vintage said, "Pain has become my constant companion. Pain is always with me even during the night. He requires minimal attention, has few demands, and I can always count on his being with me no matter where I am!"

I have become a creature of habit. I find myself less and less interested in doing new things. What a difference from that former Marilyn who would jump on a plane in a heartbeat to travel to a new place. I still drive, but only to familiar places. Jumping into a car and crossing the country is a thing of the past.

Gloria Steinem is one of my heroes. I have always admired her courage and energy that helped change the world. In 1984, tired of all the, "You don't look your age!" remarks she famously said, "This is what 50 looks like!" pointing to herself. Many women in those days primped themselves to please and pamper men so they considered "You don't look your age" a compliment. Gloria refused to accept such a compliment and told the media why.

I agree that women should not be rated solely on their looks. Neither should men. But we live in a visual world. At this writing the hair styles of female TV journalists remind me of a spaniel's ears. But I rate all journalists on their work and hair styles change as quickly as I wrinkle.

Seriously, it can be difficult to tell a person's age. So many variables! Genes, health, luck, spas, makeup, hair dye, plastic surgery, what's going in your life, what your mood is. When anyone says I look younger than my age I immediately thank the speaker. Only when I get to my mirror do I question his or her vision.

Just for fun I Googled, "What do women of 89 look like?" First, I found a bunch of photographs of old women who were missing or wanted by the law. Then there was a site with photos of women starting in their 20s but I figured it would tire this old lady out to scroll down through all those years!

Wait, my aged brain just remembered a recent compliment from a professional. My eye doctor remarked at my annual exam, "You have beautiful eyeballs. Come back in a year." Wow! Not only do I <u>not</u> have macular degeneration, thank goodness, but I have beautiful eyeballs.

I am so grateful that I still have gratitude! The man in my life, my wonderful family, and all my many friends. Every sunrise and sunset. The mountains and clouds. Music. Books. Make your own list. Every day that we oldies can add to that list is magical.

What do I regret? I once wrote that I decided to review the bad things I did in my life from disobeying the teacher in kindergarten onward. By the time I had traced my sins to about middle age, I laughed out loud! My sins were neither awful nor did I repeat them.

At this writing, I regret not being kinder. I wanted to be kind, but could have held my tongue a couple of hundred times. Obviously, sainthood is not in the cards.

What do I hope for? World peace. Survival of our beautiful, beloved Planet Earth. Schooling for all so that ignorance is conquered. The continued advancement of science and knowledge to help humankind. Support for the arts to enhance all of our lives. The survival of democracy. And a soft landing when my end approaches.

I am troubled by the divisiveness we see all over the world. My mother was alive during the War to End All Wars. I remember World War II, the establishment of the United Nations, the "One World" concept.

Years ago, my late husband and I came out of a movie that featured an Italian wedding. I mused, aloud, "That Italian wedding was so much like a Jewish wedding." He replied, "Yes, Marilyn, you see ethnicity is universal."

In a way it is. As humans evolved, it was important to recognize a tribe member. Great, this isn't an enemy. This guy can help me kill that saber-toothed tiger over there. Those tigers and other megafauna became extinct 12,000 years ago. Today's horrific threats ... nuclear war, climate change ... are not tribal, they are global. Solutions must be global.

Of course, let's enjoy and cherish our own "tribe." But let's use more of our brain than our fine-tuned facial recognition ability. Let's use the thinking parts of our brain to realize that every group is composed of people who also enjoy and cherish their own customs whether they drink Chianti or Kosher wine. My way of thinking is that we are all one people on a fragile planet. This means we have to work together to solve global problems.

When everybody feels this way, some far day in a Utopian future, we'll all drink champagne together to celebrate! L'Chaim! A toast to life!

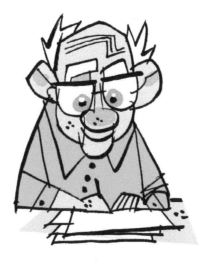

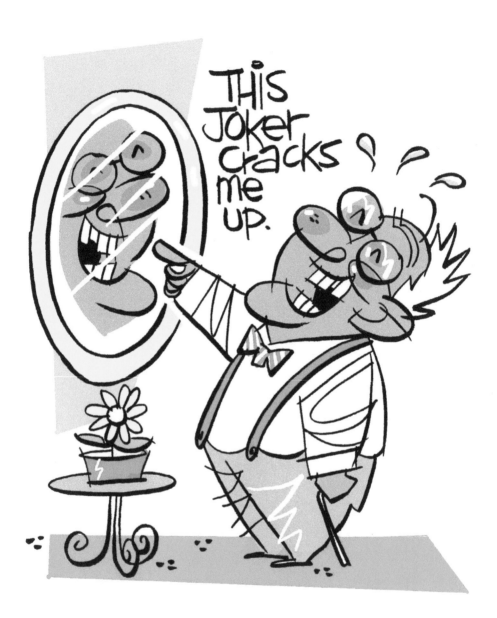

CHAPTER 16

FINDING HUMOR IN GERIATRICA

Today on our morning walk a neighbor and his wife, who had not seen me for a couple of weeks, asked where I had been. I explained my right knee was giving me trouble.

"Only ONE knee hurts?" he queried. We all burst out laughing. To those of us who live with Elderpains, it was hilarious. And factual. Our aches and pains are frequently multiple.

Why? All Darwin and Mother Nature expect of us is to pass on our genes. After that we are superfluous, so we were not designed to live to a ripe old age. In addition, many of us have lived an active life, spurred on by the media and our doctors telling us to get up off our seat and move. Some of us have played too many sets and hoisted too many pounds.

FUN FACTS ABOUT AGING

Lots of us are living to a ripe old age. In 1900, life expectancy in the United States was 47 years. It rose steadily to 78.7 although suicide and opiates are messing things up so life expectancy has decreased in the last two years. Sadly, it is also affected by household income and zip code. Poverty does not lead to a ripe old age.

Lifespan is the maximum number of years a human being can live. At this point in time the winner of the Lifespan Olympics is a French lady named Jeanne Louise Calment who died in 1997 at the age of 122 years and 164 days. She was described as being relatively "healthy and mentally intact until her 122nd birthday." An amazing woman!

The human lifespan has lengthened in industrialized nations. This happened because public health and medicine brought about good hygiene, safe water, breathable air, less crowding, immunizations, and antibiotics.

Longevity, defined as a long duration of an individual life, is becoming more common in recent years thanks to the availability of medical care and medications that cure or manage diseases like cancer or heart disease.

Yet the age to which most of us in the US can expect to live is forty-four years **younger** than the human lifespan. Scientists are working on finding a modern-day Fountain of Youth to close that gap. But for me the magic potion would have to keep me living longer and HEALTHIER.

Those of us in Geriatrica will no doubt be gone long before water from such a fountain can benefit any of us. Readers know I advise us old folks to take care of ourselves, avoid falls, and beware of loneliness. Here is a fourth bit of advice: laugh a lot about old age and anything else that tickles your funny bone. Though longevity is not dependent solely on optimism and a positive attitude, it sure can't hurt and laughing is more fun than bewailing and complaining. It has been said that laughter is the best medicine and we don't need to worry about a prescription or co-pay.

HUMOR HELPS!

Aging is no joke (although we oldies can be the butt of jokes) but laughing makes us feel good while moaning and groaning make us feel worse.

Dr. William Quinn, a fellow pediatrician, wrote in the *The American Academy of Pediatrics Senior Bulletin*, what he learned through the ages of his life. At 82, "I've learned that even when I have pains, I don't have to be one." At 92 he admits, "I've learned that I still have a lot to learn."

Will Rogers kept America laughing and had lots to say about aging though he died in a plane crash at age 56. "You know you are getting old when everything either dries up or leaks." "One must wait until evening to see how splendid the day has been." "If you don't learn to laugh at trouble, you won't have anything to laugh at when you're old."

American writer Ambrose Bierce gathered his satiric definitions into a single book, *The Devil's Dictionary*, first published in 1906 under a different title. I cannot pick up my falling-apart paperback without laughing out loud. He defines life as "... a spiritual pickle preserving the body from decay. We live in daily apprehension of its loss yet when lost it is not missed." Longevity: "Uncommon extension of the fear of death."

A delightful book by Father Gander (Douglas Larche), *Father Gander Nursery Rhymes*, brings gender equality to the nursery where it belongs. One reviewer used the term "Equal Rhymes Amendment." An example, "Jack be nimble, Jack be quick, Jack jump over the candle stick! Jill be nimble, jump it too, If Jack can do it, so can you!" (Grandparents, take note. You can entertain the young ones with such poems and teach them an important lesson at the same time.)

Musical jokes abound. Here are my two faves. Gilbert, the lyricist half of Gilbert and Sullivan, had a sharp wit and sharper tongue. When a woman, not very knowledgeable about music asked," "Is Bach still composing?" he retorted, "No, madam, he is decomposing." Fred Allen, "When Jack Benny plays the violin it sounds as if the strings are still back in the cat!"

Limericks, both clean and dirty, can make me laugh. Pick up a book of limericks at the book store or library and laugh away!

Even infirmities like hearing loss can lead to a laugh when you realize what was said and what you heard were hilariously different, sometimes so different no lady would share why she was laughing. I like clever much more than I like farce and very much more than I like cruel humor.

Quotes from women tickle my feminist funny bone. From the entertainment business came some great quips. Producer Irene Selznick, "I'd like to grow very old as slowly as possible." Actress Jeanne Moreau, "Age does not protect you from love. But love, to some extent, protects you from age." Phyllis Diller, "Never go to bed mad, stay up and fight!" Author Agatha Christie, "An archeologist is the best husband any woman can have. The older she gets, that more interested he is in her."

Although this is pretty serious, it fits perfectly in a book about aging. Elizabeth Kübler-Ross, who taught us all about death and dying, offers great advice. "The ultimate lesson all of us have to learn is **UNCONDITIONAL LOVE**, which includes not only others but ourselves as well."

Grandchildren can tickle our funny bones with their cute sayings. Lilah, age 20 months, had been taught sign language by her mom so she could communicate before she became a fluent talker. She was already bibbed and high-chaired when her mother sat down next to her at a big family gathering. Lilah immediately signed, "Wash your hands first!" If she was able to correctly correct her mother when she was a toddler, Mommy had a lot to look forward to.

Joshua, age five, was asked if he wanted ice cream. "No, Daddy, I have no room. I'll eat it when the food in my stomach goes down to my poop." A budding physiologist?

Joshua and Mom were stuck in LA traffic trying to get to school. Frazzled Mom, "Maybe we should move our house closer to the school." Joshua thought a moment and then said, "I don't think that will work, Mommy. The house is too heavy and it's stuck to the ground." Maybe an engineer?

A message for my fellow dwellers in Geriatrica: A house that rings with laughter, or even a few chuckles or giggles, is healthy. It's one of the best ways to turn off that sad or worried tape playing in your head.

YOUR MAP

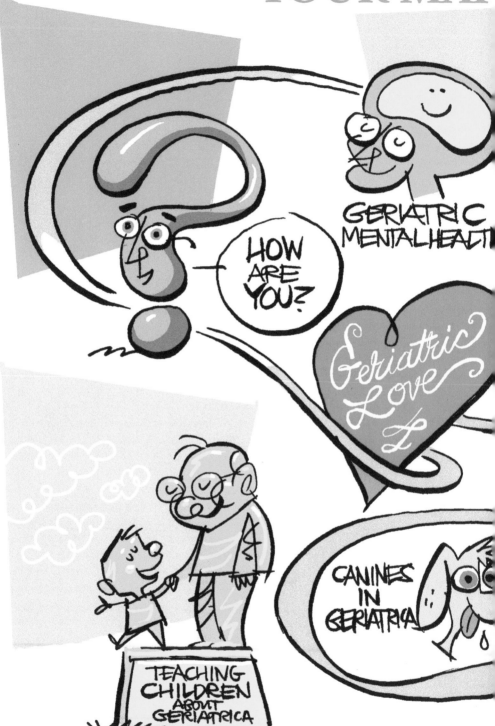

FOR PART III

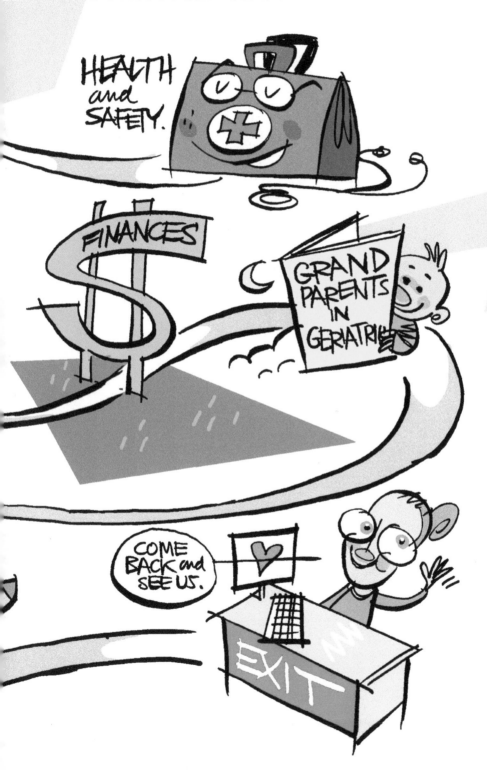

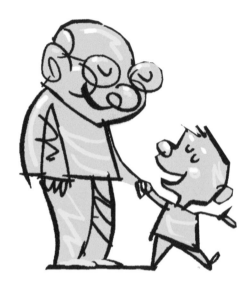

PART III INTRODUCTION

INFORMATION ABOUT YOUR NEW LAND

These chapters will help you focus on how to deal with the tasks of settling down in your new land. You will learn how to take care of your health and mental health and ways to answer questions about how you are doing here. You will read about geriatric love and finances, always compelling subjects. Next is information on the roles of grandparents in Geriatrica and how to teach young children about your new land. There is a chapter on canines who dwell here and how they can help us. And even a chapter on COVID-19 invading the land of Geriatrica.

The last chapter is a summing up chapter entitled CODA.

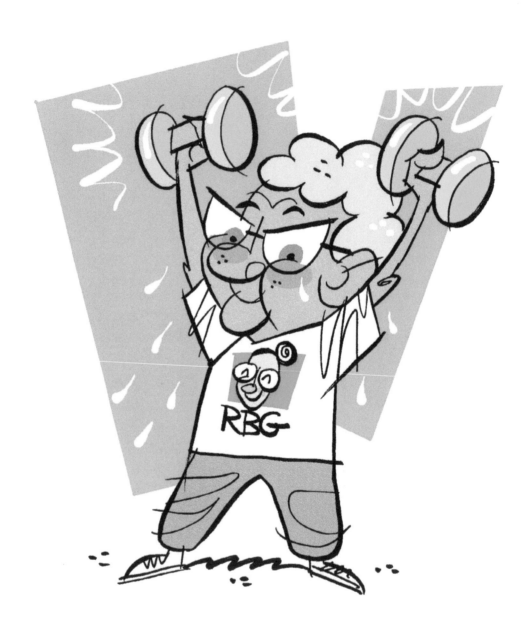

CHAPTER 17

GERIATRIC HEALTH AND SAFETY

I am a pediatrician, a parenting-through-the-life-cycle columnist, an avid reader about health issues, and an octogenarian. Does that make me qualified to write about health issues in the geriatric crowd? You be the judge.

Aging brings about many wear and tear problems to virtually all of us. Arthritic joints, fragile skin, diminishing eyesight and hearing, balance problems, memory loss, crumbling teeth, etc. All these symptoms are very common. They occur because we were lucky enough to have survived to old age and our body is wearing out. Just think of the number of times we have used our thumbs or knees, the wonderful places we have walked. No wonder these joints have become arthritic!

Our goal as residents of Geriatrica is to maintain the highest quality of health possible. Hopefully, because we are in our new land, we were dealt good genes including at least one for longevity. Thank you, Mom and Dad!

PREVENTION

Genes are not enough. We also have to take care of ourselves. I once wrote, "Longevity depends on genes and luck but we have to give prevention a chance." We must parent ourselves as there is nobody around to say, Eat your vegetables or Wash your hands.

Get ALL the recommended immunizations, stay as active and mobile as you can be, and wash your hands with soap after using the toilet, when you come back to the house, and before handling food. I know that is many times during the day ... and night, I have an old bladder too!

Eat healthy without being fanatic about food. I know many "Food Phobics." They once read something that warned red meat or butter were harmful and fear this foodstuff forever, even if the science has changed. Remember when we were all told to eat margarine, butter was bad? Then butter won out. Fear of food is foolish unless there is an allergy or food intolerance. Balance is important when it comes to both diets and preventing falls.

Michael Pollan wrote this sensible recipe for eating healthy, "Eat food, not too much, mostly plants." Food means real food and avoiding "edible food-like substances ... with 15 ingredients you can't pronounce." He means precooked or prepackaged food. I confess to having some on hand for emergencies but I treat them like candy. My mother said I could have candy once in a while, but not every day and I have lived to be 90.

I found it difficult to cook for one person after my husband died. My solution was to always cook for two or more meals. Leftovers work for me because they are less work. Not cooking at all is also an option, especially in hot weather, so I eat lots of salads, and turn some leftovers into sandwiches.

Be sure to eat enough. Geriatricians point out it's better to have a bit of fat on your bones than to look like a stick. Why? Because if you become ill or have to be hospitalized this gives you a cushion. (No pun intended.)

When people live alone it can be a challenge to remember mealtimes and shopping is sometimes difficult for us oldies. Plan ahead to ensure your cupboard is not bare. Ask friends or neighbors to help in a pinch.

Avoid falls. They can be lethal or life-altering. According to the *Journal of the American Medical Association* they are increasing in frequency as we oldies increase. Health care cost from fatal and nonfatal falls? About 50 billion dollars.

Remember childproofing the house when your baby started to crawl? Same principle: push chairs under the table, eliminate scatter rugs, be sure there is adequate lighting and night lights that go on automatically. I keep a flashlight in my nightstand and in other key places in case of a power failure.

Common sense stuff: Smoke and carbon monoxide detectors are a must. If one goes off or you smell smoke, you and your loved ones including pets should leave the house immediately. Don't wait to save possessions, you are the irreplaceable one.

If you have a "smart car" in an attached garage, be sure the car is completely turned off when you leave it. If not, carbon monoxide can creep into your house with fatal results. Once I inadvertently left my car on while I had a hair trim and pedicure. By the time I came out my battery was dead. I had to be rescued by AAA.

Stoves and refrigerators can be dangerous to your health. Be sure the stove is OFF. Beware of spoiled food. Use the Sniff Test on any food item that, like us oldies, is beyond its original prime. Also refrigerate perishables quickly and do not leave food out in the sun or the heat.

Speaking of sun and heat, use sunscreen, dress cool and wear a hat. Keep yourself well hydrated, and remember Noel Coward's song that tells you only mad dogs and Englishmen go out in the noonday sun.

Finally, do all you can to prevent or avoid loneliness and social isolation. Both are associated with a decline in physical and mental health and premature death. Being alone can lead to impaired mobility, chronic illness, and cognitive decline as well as depression. If circumstances have dealt you the living alone card, do all you can to get out of the house, make new friends, and be active in all ways you can be. Consider a senior facility sooner rather than later before you are afflicted with any of the above. (See Chapter 5.)

DOCTORS

Doctors cure or try to cure diseases. They cannot cure aging.

But they can help us stay healthy, advise us how to deal with the inevitable problems of aging, and take care of us when we get sick. Provided you listen to and follow directions and take medications as directed.

Our current health care system is pretty good for those of us on Medicare although the cost of prescription drugs is still a huge problem in this country. Many drug plans go out to recess after a certain ceiling has been reached.

I just read a bulletin from the National Health Interview Survey on strategies people over 65 use to reduce prescription drug costs. Five percent did not take medicine as directed and 18 percent asked their doctor for a lower cost alternative. Those with Medicare only (could not afford supplemental insurance) were the most likely to not take medications prescribed. Money talks, but what it says to people in poverty is not printable.

Many areas are dealing with a shortage of primary care doctors ... the internists, geriatricians, and family practitioners we go to for our annual physical or when we have a problem.

Every one of us should have a primary care doctor. If you don't, find one as soon as you can. How? Word of mouth from friends is helpful. Some doctors have waiting lists for new patients. Sign up right away as the list gets longer every day.

Think of your doctor as your partner. Don't be a silent partner. You know yourself and your body better than anybody else does. Tell your doctor what's going on.

Don't play doctor. Distinguished physician Sir William Osler said, "A physician who treats himself has a fool for a patient."

Keep track. Write down any problems you are having before you go to the doctor. I do an assessment of me before I go to the doctor. I evaluate myself from my head to my feet, the way I was taught in medical school to do a "review of systems" on patients. From this list I decide what has changed or what is now bothering me.

I take this list to my doctor and jot down what she says about each problem. Also take a list of your medications, both prescription and over-the-counter. (This list with the names of all your doctors, as well as next of kin information, should be in your wallet at all times as emergencies do happen.)

I keep a medical file on myself. After every doctor visit I file the summary my doctor gives me along with the Medication Information sheets on any new drugs prescribed. I glance at this file before I go to my doctor or another health professional like a dentist or a medical specialist so I can fill out the health questionnaires they usually ask for. I also file results of lab tests and X-rays.

Doctors have their own language and often speak in initials as a short cut. Good docs usually translate for you but if not, ASK! A friend was discharged from the hospital where she was treated for pneumonia. She was called by her doctor's office after a follow-up X-ray was read and told her chest was "clear." My friend had expected to hear her pneumonia was better and, though it was, she still worried because nobody said that. "What does that mean?" are four little words to use when we do not understand a health professional.

Fortunately we don't catch a cold every few weeks like kids do but we sure can be laid low by pneumonia, shingles, or flu all of which can be prevented or made less deadly by immunizations. Keep all of your immunizations up to date and file the information. Once upon a time, which I actually remember, there was nothing doctors could do for most infectious diseases of childhood. I had them all except for polio. Remember the treatment and prevention of infectious diseases is one of the reasons for our longevity.

Many surgical procedures and medications that save lives today were not invented or perfected when I was in practice. Diseases of the heart or cancer or painful hips and other joints can strike and may require a referral to a specialist. Sometimes after treatment you will be referred back to your primary care doctor or the specialist may still want to see you. If you continue to see both the specialist (or several specialists) as well as your primary, make sure that ALL know about ALL of your medications, including over-the-counter stuff.

One question I get from parents of young children AND the elderly is, "When should I call the doctor?"

Most of us know what a medical emergency is (the sudden

onset of difficulty breathing, loss of consciousness, collapse, uncontrolled bleeding, trouble speaking or moving, chest pain, seizures). And we know how to call 911.

By the way, if you feel you need to go to the hospital and there is no one to drive you, call 911. One feisty 75-year-old lady I know was having severe dizzy spells so she drove herself to the hospital. She made it but this was NOT a good idea. Think of the consequences if you were to hit somebody or a tree.

What about when you feel sick and wonder whether you need a doctor? I taught parents to use the "Three Ps" to decide when to take the child to the doctor. This strategy applies to you too. The first P stands for Personal Pattern. Do you always cough like this when you get a cold or is this a cough like you never had before? The second P is Persistence. Does the pain you felt in your wrist after typing for a couple of hours go away or does it stick around? The third P is Progression. Is the symptom getting worse?

If you are in doubt, see a doctor. I was once miserable with a fever but did not think I needed a trip to the ER. I took Tylenol and went to an Urgent Care Center when it opened in the morning. I was diagnosed with Influenza A and treated there with Tamiflu. I called my own doctor to make a follow-up appointment. The flu made me the sickest I ever felt so I am glad I could get help quickly. Lest you think I neglected myself, I did get a "high-test" flu shot but it was a year that the strain of flu I had was not protected against.

Don't believe all you read on the Internet. I always felt uncomfortable answering a parent's medical question online without examining the child. I told parents I could give generic advice about an illness but for prescription advice, the child had to be seen. That goes for us elderfolk too.

It's OK to use the Internet to get general information provided you go to a reputable source. However, try to protect yourself from Medical Student Sickness which is feeling symptoms of every disease you are currently studying.

An online list of all the symptoms caused, for example, by a medication you are reading about can make you reluctant to take the medication. These lists can describe a symptom reported by a fairly small number of people in the original studies of effectiveness or by doctors after the drug is on the market. They are of interest but usually rare. Your doctor knows about these side effects before Mr. Google does. Listen to your doctor who weighs harm from your disease against harm from the drug.

Sometimes the Medication Information sheet says, "Do not discontinue the medication without calling your doctor." This is very important because it can be dangerous to stop it abruptly. Sometimes it reads, "If X occurs, stop the medication and call your doctor immediately." Best you call your physician if you have any symptoms that started after you started a medication.

Just yesterday I was asked how do you navigate today's health care system. "I had surgery that did not relieve my symptoms and I want to see another specialist." My advice, "Call your primary care doctor to answer this question." Reading online a list of specialists and how they were rated will not help you. Like children you need specific not generic advice. Five stars will not tell you if this is the specialist you need. Plus your insurance may require you choose from a specific list of doctors or you will not be reimbursed.

If you seek specific medical information about yourself but are not sick, call the doctor. Many doctors today are also available on the office website and a non-emergency medical question will be answered within 48 hours.

If you feel sick and want to be seen, call your doctor. Often you will be asked to speak to the doctor's assistant first who will convey your symptoms to the doctor and call you back if you need to be seen. Sometimes the assistant will suggest what you can try to avoid a visit.

Finally, be a good patient. Compliant, but able to speak up for yourself if necessary. For example, you have a respiratory infection and were told it needed no treatment but now you are having pain every time you take a deep breath. Your doctor needs to know this. Don't forget to be polite and respectful to the office staff. They have a tough job too, especially when the office is busy.

On a personal note, I told my doctor I hope I expire before she retires! Doctors need to be told how much they are appreciated.

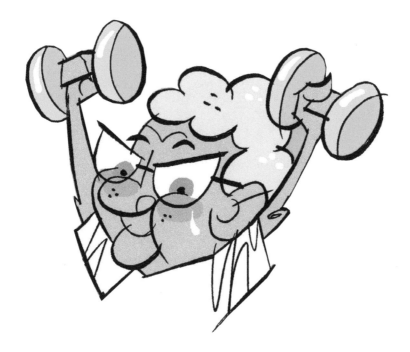

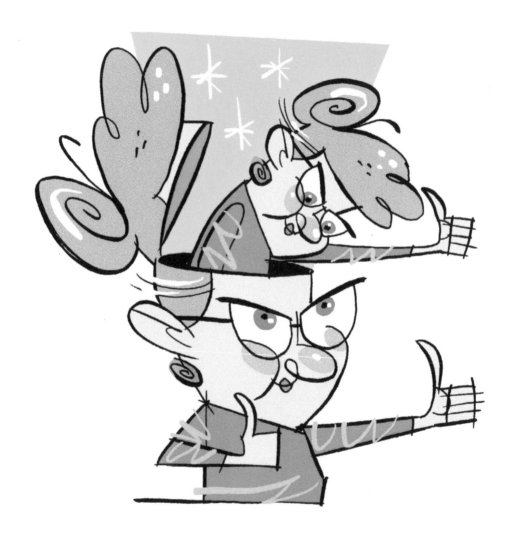

CHAPTER 18

GERIATRIC MENTAL HEALTH

Mental health in the aged is a serious problem. World population is aging rapidly and is predicted to rise from 12 percent in 2015 to almost 22 percent by 2050. Approximately 15 percent of the aged worldwide have a mental health disorder. As the U.S. population ages it is estimated as many as 20 percent of people age 55 years or older will suffer from a mental health concern or condition. That's one out of five of us.

The most prevalent geriatric mental health problems are depression (and its twin, anxiety) and dementia. Everybody, old or young, will feel very sad or terribly anxious or awfully upset because they can't remember something sometime. But the two big bad Ds ... dementia and depression ... are real diseases affecting the brain. They both are life-altering.

DEMENTIA

There are several causes of dementia including early onset Alzheimer's, Alzheimer's disease (AD), Lewy body dementia, frontotemporal dementia, Parkinson's disease, vascular cognitive impairment, traumatic brain injury, Huntington's disease, and others. Some dementias caused by vitamin deficiencies or infections can be somewhat reversed, but most cannot. The saddest dementia is early onset Alzheimer's disease because it attacks people well before old age.

The most common (70 percent) is Alzheimer's disease. The Alzheimer's Association projects that by 2030 the number of those with AD will more than double and by 2050 may grow from 5.5 million to 13.8 million, barring medical breakthroughs to "prevent, slow, or cure" this scourge. The lifetime risk for getting this disease is 11.6 percent for males and 21.1 percent for females. The estimated cost of caring for these patients is astronomical.

There is a genetic component to AD that has been known and studied for many years. But having this factor does not mean you will get Alzheimer's and not having it will not prevent it. Much work remains to be done on this.

Can we predict AD? A recent study found that there was a link between those who fell for a scam, like the IRS calling to say you owe them money that must be sent immediately, and the development of AD. (See Chapter 3, Scams Designed Just for You.)

Almost 100 percent of us old folks will exhibit some signs of what is called minimal cognitive impairment (MCI). There are jokes about us being forgetful, absent minded, losing things. This comes with our new territory. If you are worried, your primary care doctor can administer a short mental status exam that, hopefully, will alleviate your worries.

The symptoms of AD may appear slowly. They include progressive memory loss, decline in visual/spatial abilities, trouble with problem solving, difficulties with complex tasks, coordination and motor problems, confusion. The person may repeat a question several times or agree to a suggestion but quickly forget it. And may wander off and not be able to get back home. Confusion and frustration can sometimes lead to violence. Judgment is affected.

Obviously when the diagnosis of AD is made, family members must make a plan to take over medications, finances, and do all they can to prevent an AD victim from doing things dangerous to self or others. Memory Care facilities may be needed, especially if the patient is a wanderer.

There are also psychological symptoms like personality changes, depression, anxiety, paranoia, agitation, hallucinations. I remember a friend with AD I picked up and took out for lunch.

When her coffee was poured, she opened up all the little creamers on the table one at a time and put them all in her coffee, not noticing the cup began to overflow.

Some of these cognitive or personality changes are noticed by a spouse or relative before the person is aware of what is going on. Patients with dementia may say things like, "I don't know what to do with this," holding out a familiar object, or, "I can't remember how to turn my computer on." They may look bewildered or puzzled in a place they had been to many times. They may be so frustrated that they become violent. Or so frightened they refuse to leave their still familiar chair.

At this point in time we cannot prevent or cure Alzheimer's although many research efforts are underway. Without question it's healthy for us oldies to keep our minds and bodies active. But no matter how many crossword puzzles we do or power walks we take, sadly we could be stricken. This scourge comes with aging. There are some medications that may delay worsening of dementia but there is as yet no cure. Support AD research!

DEPRESSION

Depression is a medical condition of the brain that is treatable, like diabetes or hypertension. It can run in families. Symptoms include feelings of sadness or anxiety that do not go away. Persons who are depressed have feelings of hopelessness or pessimism. They may feel worthless, helpless, irritable or demonstrate restlessness, fatigue, loss of energy, difficulty concentrating or making decisions. There may be sleep problems from insomnia to excessive sleep or appetite changes from eating very little to using food to dull the pain. Physical symptoms like aches or pains or digestive symptoms are fairly common. Thoughts of suicide or attempts are an indication of the seriousness of depression.

Many or most people with depression also suffer anxiety. Anxiety is a normal and healthy emotion that has helped humankind survive. Hearing a saber-toothed tiger growling meant danger. Danger scares us and fear starts a rush of adrenalin that reacts in what is called a "fight-or-flight" response. Our heart beats faster so we can escape.

But the anxiety of depression can take over your life with uncontrollable feelings of worry. It's like a tape playing in your heard that doesn't stop. One person I know described her symptoms concisely, "I am sad and scared all the time!" Fear can lead to not leaving the house and being housebound, especially if you live alone, can make you sadder.

Many of us have experienced symptoms of depression when grieving the loss of a loved one. I flew home alone after my husband's funeral in another state. I could remember nothing of the trip, though I had managed to get home by myself.

The next morning ... and for many mornings ... I awoke with an enormous sense of a loss that was permanent and irrevocable. This caused such deep and bleak grief that I wanted to pull the sheets over my head and stay in bed forever. Luckily I had a dog who rarely barked but somehow knew barking was now essential to get me out of bed and on the other end of her leash. I also sought and greatly profited by talk therapy.

Older adults are at increased risk for depression as it is more common in people who also have other illnesses (such as heart disease or cancer) or whose life becomes limited from the aging process. About 80 percent of older adults have at least one chronic health condition, and 50 percent have two or more. An elderly person living alone, especially a man, has an increased risk for dying prematurely.

Depression can be greatly helped or totally reversed with medication. If any readers out there are worried about depression symptoms, start with a visit to your primary care doctor.

This is the person to help you sort out your symptoms and decide whether you need treatment. The doctor will help you decide between medications and counseling or both. And make referrals for psychiatric admission if necessary. Talk to your doctor sooner not later. Suffering in silence is not the way to live your golden years. By the way, grief-caused depression hurts as much as any depression. And if it lingers or worsens it may need the same treatment ranging from talk therapy to medication or both.

Depression is very real and very painful and can be fatal. It can also be cured or greatly ameliorated. I grew up at a time when mental illness was shameful and concealed. Fortunately times have changed. One can talk about depression today and there are also some strategies we can do for ourselves. Exercise really helps, as does keeping busy.

Longevity means losses, but the loss of our mind due to dementia or the ravaging of our moods due to depression, is dreadful to both endure or contemplate.

If you or a loved one have symptoms of either dementia or depression, don't suffer in silence or wait for such these symptoms to go away, Get help! If depression strikes, be thankful there is help. If dementia is diagnosed, difficult as this will be for both you and your family, planning for the future can begin.

CAREGIVERS

A postscript for caregivers. Mental illness in a loved one affects the entire family. In my age group a typical family consists of a person living alone or two people aging together. Two people is better and actually healthier, but when one develops a mental illness, two people suffer.

If a partner seems depressed be understanding and supportive but do all you can to see that he or she gets help. Saying, "Snap out of it!" does not work.

My late husband died of Alzheimer's dementia. We both suffered. I was fortunate to be able to hire help but running a one-bed nursing home for three years was the hardest task of my life. The only way I could survive was to get individual and group therapy help for myself.

If you are such a caregiver remember the flight attendant's words: "If you are travelling with an infant put the mask on yourself first and then help the baby." The message is clear: without oxygen you cannot save the baby. Without help for yourself, you cannot help your loved one.

BAD, SAD DAYS

What can we do to keep our spirits up as we age? Because longevity means losses, it is likely we will all have bad, sad days.

We can count and know our days are numbered. They are when we are young too, but youth comes with built-in optimism that often dwindles as we age.

These bad, sad days may not be clinical depression, but they sure can feel like it.

Here is a list of what I do to recover from such a day.

1. My mother had a friend who would say, "Why speak of it?" when bad, sad thoughts arose.

2. Why even think of it? Shake off these thoughts that creep up unawares. Pretend you are a dog shaking off water from its back.

3. Telling your thoughts to shut up is a difficult task. But doing something active like taking a walk or going to the gym can help.

4. To "treat" a bad day I have a routine I do. I make myself go through the motions of my day, get out of the house, do some exercise, call somebody. And if I get through the day, I give myself a little victory present like a piece of chocolate and pat myself on the head. I can't reach my back any more.

5. If it's a bad day for a reason like the anniversary of a loved one's death or birthday, wallow in your grief. Cry, look at pictures, remember the person. But just for one day. Remember the five-second rule? Make wallowing a one-day rule.

I am still alive thanks to scientific Western Medicine. But Eastern Medicine has some useful methods that can prevent and help with sad, bad days as well as chronic pain. Yoga, meditation, Tai Chi, acupuncture, mindfulness, massage can work wonders. Don't use in place of going to a doctor, consider it supplemental. East and West working together!

There are some self-help strategies I use. Seeing and keeping in touch with younger friends helps me. During lunch with one of my dear friends young enough to be my daughter, she used the phrase "textured friendships" to describe interactions with people of all ages. Nice description! I reach out to my younger friends and find them exhilarating. No, I cannot keep up with them but hearing about their work, projects, travels is like a tonic. Another way to lift my spirits is taking courses at the university. Seeing younger people and exercising my brain makes me feel (almost) young again!

The Harvard School of Public Health published the results of a study that showed optimists live longer. An optimist believes good things will happen while pessimists always see the future as bleak. We always figured people came that way, either optimistic or pessimistic. But maybe we can find ways to modulate these traits.

Some years ago, my daughter gave me a sweet little dish only big enough to hold a ring or two. Painted in bright colors, it reads," I think I will just be happy today." Why not?

And maybe, just maybe, if we decided to be happy **every day**, our bad, sad, pessimistic days would diminish!

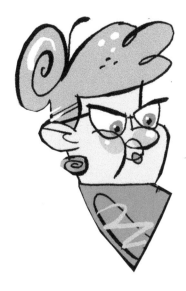

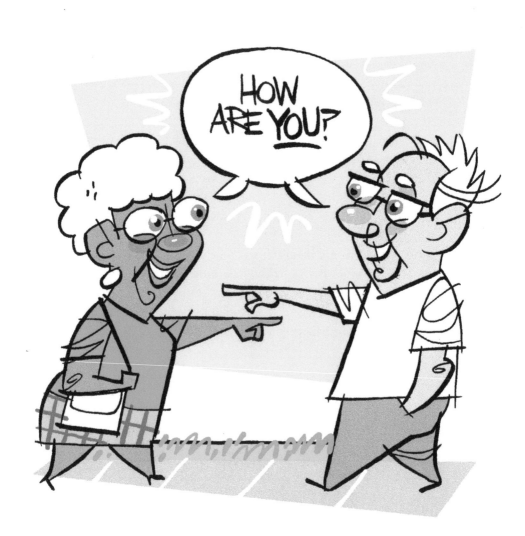

CHAPTER 19

ANSWERS TO "HOW ARE YOU?"

What should we old folks answer when we meet a friend who asks, "How are you?"

"Fine! How are you?" was my routine answer when I was young. Those of us in what I call Advanced Old Age must now decide how to best deal with this simple question.

Remember losing and forgetting things goes with the territory in Geriatrica. One witty man I know told me that instead of those tiny spaces between his brain neurons, his synapses were now filled with molasses. That is why it takes so long for a memory to be remembered.

Do we play the martyr and through clenched teeth and a forced wan smile caused by our cranky knee tell a big lie, "Fine, fine, how are you?"

Do we make a lame joke? "I'm aging, thank you!" "I must be OK, I woke up on the right side of the grass this morning!" "I am vertical and still ventilating!" "Not bad for an old geezer!" "I am surprised I'm still here!" "Why complain, nobody wants to hear it?"

(I refrain from saying, "The old, grey Mare-ilyn ain't what she used to be!")

Or do we tell the truth? A litany of nonstop truth like, "I feel awful, my back is killing me, I am uncomfortable day and night even with an expensive new mattress, the doctor said there is nothing she can do, I cut my finger peeling an onion. I am depressed and irritable, etc. etc." Boring!

My favorite answer comes from a dear lady with several health issues, but nonetheless a sunny and optimistic outlook. When I ask how she is, her answer is, "Fabulous and YOU look fabulous too!"

My advice is to be truthful but not ruin anybody's day. I might say something like, "I am getting physical therapy for my sore neck and it seems to be helping." But I will not list all the things that bother or worry me. Friends have much better things to talk about!

When our children ask how we are, what do we say? My children, none of whom live nearby, call me almost every day. We mostly talk about what is going on, what movies we saw or books we read. I relish little anecdotes about the grandchildren or news of their accomplishments.

They ask how I am doing and I try not to complain. They have their own children, their own worries. None of us wants to be a "problem case" for our children.

However, when we reach Geriatrica, our children will worry. They feel 1. We do or may soon need their help in dealing with a major health problem. 2. They are concerned we may not be able to manage on our own.

If they live far away, it can make the worry worse. It certainly made me worry a lot about my mother who lived in Massachusetts, kitty corner away from Arizona on a map of our very big country.

If they live nearby, they have to figure out how to best help you without interfering with your autonomy. How to best deal with "reverse parenting," my term for the state of affairs when the children must step in for your health and safety.

Remember, we had to step in for safety 's sake when our child needed supervision. We tried to dance between living their lives for them and giving them the space to become a grownup.

I have never concealed facts about my health from my children. They deserve to know the truth. And if the time comes when they have to step in and "reverse parent" me I will try to be gracious, a good role model for them to remember when they grow old.

Facts. Those of us who live in Geriatrica are growing old, the opposite of growing up. The incurable and unstoppable process called aging brings changes in our bodies that cannot be reversed. Even a vegan who runs a marathon every week will age!

The issue is how much do we want to talk about our aging processes? Does it help to talk about such problems? Sometimes. Will it bore your friends and children to tears? Sometimes. If you conceal facts or cover up problems will children and friends get mad? Probably.

Most of us in advanced old age have signs of what I call Elderbrain, Elderbalance, Elderjoints, and Elderbladder. I have symptoms of all of these. Though my expertise is in Babybrain and Babybladder, I have lots of personal experience in Elderwhatever. Enough to write a book!

But I get angry with myself when I dwell on these facts of my new life in Geriatrica. For example, the retrieval time to bring a fact I know out of the depths can be long enough to infuriate me because I know I know it, darn it!

Lost items can be a challenge? I have learned that, when I cannot find where I put something in my own house, swearing and getting cross with myself is counterproductive. I go to a comfortable chair, close my eyes, relax and hum music or recite poetry to myself. It works most of the time. When I am calm instead of frantic, I may remember the route I took when I put object X in place X. If it doesn't work, the object is either gone forever or the Goddess Serendipity will lead me to it one day. By the way if you lose your car keys, wags tell us this does not mean dementia. But if you forget what they are for it is nature's way of telling us to stop driving!

I am grateful for my mobility, creaky as it is. But I figure every joint in my body has ached one time or another and we have 360 joints!

I try to walk and do exercises daily. My doctor, physical

therapist, and personal trainer all say the same thing: keep moving! My therapist said it is better to ache a bit when exercising than to become immobile from lack of exercise.

Just the other day I worried about future immobility and envisioned myself bent over leaning on a walker. My mood plummeted from neutral to sad. Then I had the jolt of an optimistic thought: If I ever do need a walker, I will paint it a bright, shiny red with sequins and flaunt it! Maybe even start a Red Walker Club!

And just about all old folks have Elderbladders. Very few of us sleep through the night without our bladder alarm going off and waking us. We stagger to the bathroom (night lights are a must!) and if we are lucky fall back to sleep quickly. When one has elderbladder it is useful to memorize the location of restrooms everywhere in your town.

Fortunately, one can have all of the elder-problems above and still lead a pretty good life. I do. My challenge is to continue doing some (not all) of the things I love without wearing myself out and to balance my life so I have enough down time. And to accept myself for who I am now, creaky knees and all!

So how much of all this geezer-complaining do our children, friends, neighbors, the postman want to hear? Should hear? Need to hear?

The answer is a combination of common sense, good manners, and boundaries. Moderation in all things.

Some of us are more reluctant to share details of our bodily failings than others are. There is a fine line between blabbing every detail at a dinner party and withholding information from an old friend.

Each of us has to decide where we are on this line. I favor telling rather than concealing the truth. Then quickly change the subject.

There are better things for us to talk about than bladders!

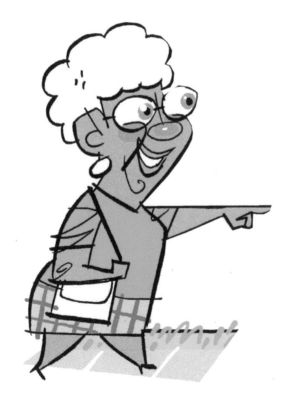

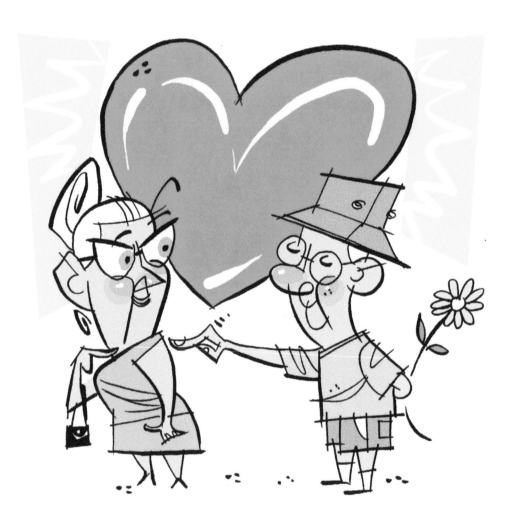

CHAPTER 20

GERIATRIC LOVE

Love in the late decades may be the last aspect of human sexuality to come out of the closet. Society accepts that not everybody is heterosexual, and the alphabet of accepted sexual preferences lengthens.

Sexuality in the elderly? Eldersex? Formerly unthinkable therefore nonexistent. Women live longer than men so such couples were rare. Freud suggests that children cannot picture their own parents having sex. (Try to picture it yourself.)

Some couples are blessed with both longevity and continuing intimacy ... they have been described as the happy few. And as some men age, they seek out younger women for rejuvenation if not true romance.

There is a curiosity about the matter of geriatric love. "Will you still need me, Will you still feed me, When I'm ninety-four?" The young Beatles were spot on in worrying about this matter.

Physicality in Geriatrica dwellers is unthinkable or laughable to many. One of my favorite quotes from a friend when asked what it is like to take her clothes off at her advanced age: "We practice MAD ... mutually assured delusion." Much better than that term we oldies remember from the Cold War days: mutually assured destruction.

We all need to love and be loved from birth to age 100 and beyond. From our first breath to the last. Gestures of love like hugs, valentines, and flowers are always appreciated.

Those of us who live in a youth culture where young bodies are worshiped can't help but notice that we no longer have such a body. When we are widowed, we wonder about a romantic future. After catching a glimpse of our varied saggings, we likely sigh and tell ourselves to forget about it.

However geriatric love, like longevity, is becoming more common. The population ages and we stay healthier longer, so there are more potential mates out there. Some meet in independent or assisted living facilities. Some meet in classes, the gym, at volunteer activities or church. Others meet the old-fashioned way, they are introduced by mutual friends. Still others meet the modern way, online.

This can be quite successful. It was for a college friend of mine whose husband left her for another woman. He changed his mind and begged her to let him come back but she threw him out. Her children and stepchildren were so angry they got together and pretended they were their mother on a dating site. Whatever they wrote worked. Their mother and her new love have been together for over 20 years.

I was married for 47 years and lived alone for six years. Love in my future? Impossible! Falling in love when you are 82 years old? Ridiculous! Meeting a mate in Geriatrica? Not bloody likely!

But geriatric love did happen to me, a totally unexpected blessing. I was a widow; my husband had died almost seven years earlier. I was resigned to live the rest of my life alone as many women do. This happens following the higher death rate in men and the fact that men generally marry younger women.

The Arizona Daily Star that has published my columns since 1989 played a major role in my good fortune. Editor Maria Parham, now retired, and I were having lunch. She mentioned a man at her church who had recently lost his wife and seemed lost himself. Maria suggested we two would be very compatible as both of us liked music, reading, cinema, theater. She said, "Let me invite you both to dinner." I replied, "No, that's for 40 year olds, give me his email address."

I sent an email: "I have known Maria for many years and value both her friendship and judgment. She said you loved music and are intelligent, thoughtful and a good conversationalist." We exchanged information about ourselves and found we liked the same music and books to an amazing degree of coincidence. He invited me to dinner (which he cooked ... a good sign from the beginning!).

Our friendship clicked. We rapidly became romantically attracted. I was a bit hesitant as things were happening too fast. But he wrote me a beautiful poem. That did it. I was smitten.

Family obligations kept us separated for several weeks. He was in Colorado, I was in Tucson. We talked every day and emailed like crazy. I flew to my daughter's home in Michigan to keep an eye on the teenage twins while she and her husband were in Europe. My new love called every day. I overheard my grandson tell his mom, "They talk for hours on the phone every day just like teenagers!"

We have been together over seven years now and feel blessed to have each other.

One of the most difficult problems was what word to use to describe our relationship.

According to Elizabeth Weil in the *New York Times*, "Until the 1970s, the American faux spouse was too rare and taboo to even try to track. In 1980, the United States Census Bureau made its first attempt at naming these creatures in order to count them. It really outdid itself lexicographically: 'person of opposite sex sharing living quarters,' abbreviated to POSSLQ and pronounced 'possle cue.'"

This may work for the Census Bureau but certainly does not work for today's geriatric couple who live together but are not married.

Companion? That's what we call well-trained dogs. Significant other? Other what? Partner? They have those at Goldman Sachs. Cohabiters? Dreadful word. My boyfriend? To introduce a nonagenarian? Ridiculous!

We settled on "Entwined." We consider ourselves and our lives entwined together." I wear an infinity ring made of entwined gold bands. We had a "Ceremony of Entwinement." Just the two of us. Outdoors watching the sun's last rays lighting the Catalina Mountains we read the commitment vows we had written to each other and watched the moon rise.

I have two children, two stepsons, four grandchildren, and two great-grandchildren. He has three children and four grand-children. None of these live in Arizona. I have already told you I refer to us as "geriatric orphans," the term I use to define old folks who must get on a plane to visit their family. Many visits in both directions have taken place. All the children have warmly accepted our relationship and they have all met each other.

Our combined ages at this writing are 97 + 90 = 187 years, almost two centuries! We both have medical issues, but they are so far under control as we are in the care of good doctors who prescribe proper medications that help what ails us ... at least to date. Because love includes paying attention, as we grow old we must be aware and keep track of each other's health and health care.

We both wear glasses and hearing aids, and we religiously pop our prescription pills. We consider ourselves lucky to be in reasonable health for our ages. We are both mobile, still drive, and have most, or at least some, of our marbles.

What about living and housing patterns of geriatric lovers? One couple travels together and see each other often, but do not live together. Another couple alternate whose house they sleep in. I even know a couple that live on different continents, but see each other often collecting many airline mileage points doing so.

We heard a lecture by neurosurgeon Allen Hamilton on the neuroscience of love. He showed us slides of brains that lit up when people were shown pictures of loved ones during brain imaging. Love depends on several brain neurotransmitters and hormones. Without getting too scientific, one of these, oxytocin (referred to as the "cuddle hormone"), not only maintains love but is healthy for us. And, listen up! We can boost our oxytocin levels by a mere seven long hugs a day. No prescription needed! No age limit!

Speaking of age, at the *Arizona Star*'s retirement party for Maria Parham, she mentioned how gratifying it was to keep in touch with reporters who met at the *Star*, married, and had children. (StarBabies?) She then said she had introduced Marilyn and Milt, pointing to us in the audience. "They thought it over very carefully but decided not to have any children!" Much laughter.

As a romantic young adolescent, I read a poem by W. B. Yeats called "When You Are Old." It begins, "When you are old and grey and full of sleep, and nodding by the fire, take down this book" and ends "One man loved the pilgrim soul in you and loved the sorrows of your changing face." I though this was the most romantic poem I had ever read.

My late husband read this to me on our fortieth anniversary and I wept. When I told this to my new love he wrote a poem for me containing the lines. "I will revive your pilgrim soul, and love the sorrows in your aging face."

Imagine how wonderful it is to know that two men understood and loved my pilgrim soul.

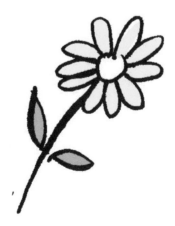

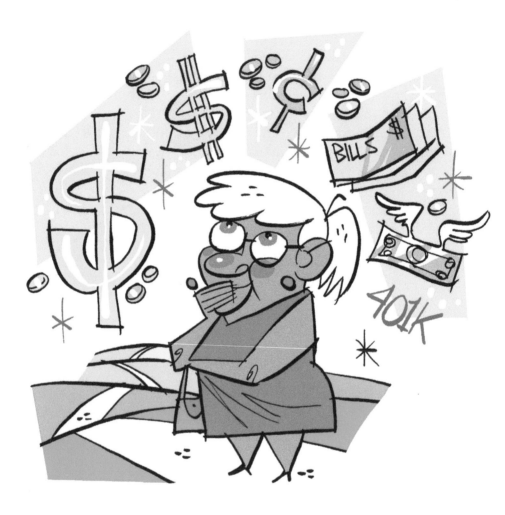

CHAPTER 21

GERIATRIC FINANCES

A complicated matter, especially for a person like me who has no head for it. I always preferred letters to numbers and reading to math.

But finances cannot be ignored because some of the important decisions we must make in our life, both before we retire and after, depend on how much money we have and whether it will last as long as we do.

Before I start, I must point out that I am writing this chapter for those fortunate people who have a pension or adequate funds in savings and/or retirement funds. I worry greatly for the many Americans who live paycheck to paycheck and weep tears of frustration about the unfair and increasing inequality in our country.

I am a retired pediatrician who was taught to stress PREVENTION, the art and science of stopping something before it happens or arises. Just as it is too late to discuss birth control with a teen who is pregnant, it is too late to think about one's financial future the day of the retirement party.

Financial planning for those living in Geriatrica, or approaching its shores, starts with asking and answering the "What if ... " questions with the family. (See Chapter 6.) What if one of you becomes ill? What if Mom dies first? Dad? What if neither of you can or want to take care of a house any longer? What if either of you needs assisted living care? Memory Care? What if neither of you can drive anymore?

Factors to be considered in planning are geography, senior facilities available, life cycle issues (a grandchild in college, a child with a chronic illness) as well as resources. These are the most hypothetical questions one can ask but do the best you can. Because any or all of these variables are likely to change, such family meetings may need to be repeated.

Both you and your children should make yourselves aware of options, facilities and eldercare services in your community. It is important to have such talks before there is a crisis, update plans periodically, and give parents as much autonomy as possible. Let me point out that not planning means someone else (or the state) will make your decisions for you. We must make sure that our wishes are written down, all legal documents are properly signed and witnessed, and are in the proper hands.

FINANCIAL PLANNING

Money matters are complicated. Especially for those of you like me who do not understand such complexities. I am fortunate to have a financial advisor whose wisdom amazes me. Over the years he has helped me make decisions to preserve my assets so I will not be a burden on my children.

He shared with me this list of mistakes he observed his senior clients make over the years.

1. One mistake is not appreciating the difference between POSSIBILITY and PROBABILITY. "It is possible the world is coming to an end. I am so scared I will do nothing." But doing nothing when it is probable the world will still be around is not a good decision because you abdicate the decision-making to circumstances. "The world is coming to an end so I will spend all my money now!" is not a cool idea because though it is possible it is not probable. The probability is that you will spend all your money and the world will go on. Now what?

2. Second, do not make financial decisions based on TV news, investment shows, or newspaper opinion pieces. Media profits by attracting people. A lurid show or scary article about stocks invokes your emotional reactions so you watch or read tomorrow.

When it comes to financial matters you should be thinking, not reacting emotionally.

3. Beware of online financial advice! I tell parents who email me for advice that I can give only "generic advice" over the Internet. If they need "prescription advice" they must take the child to a doctor. Same applies to finance.

4. Do not rely on friends, relatives or children for financial advice. You would not permit anybody but a board-certified orthopedic surgeon to operate on your hip, would you? We must rely on advice in both medical and financial matters so ask professionals.

5. Know what your annual expenditures are. Keep accurate accounts of what you spend and where your money goes. "Income can be identified by your advisors; expenditures cannot." Wise planning for the future starts with knowing what you spend now.

6. Arithmetic counts! Be accurate and sensible. A million dollars in the bank sounds pretty good. But if you have no income coming in and you spend $300,000 a year, you will probably run out of money in four years. When calculating how much spendable money your funds will generate, subtract likely taxes you will have to pay. Also factor in the increases that are likely to occur in your future care as you age.

7. Think about probable increases all possible when planning for your future. It is likely that there will be rent increases in the independent and assisted living facilities you sign up for. If you downsize to a smaller home, Home Owners Association fees will likely rise. You may still be doing house work and gardening when you move but will reach an age when you can no longer do these things. Cars and household appliances age just as we do and the costs of fixing or replacing these must be taken into account as well as our own future medical or personal care.

8. Do not give away, gift, or donate money too soon. When we are still employed or retired and comfortable it feels wonderful to lavish money on our children or make donations to worthy causes. Things can change quickly, especially our health and ability to take care of ourselves. The best inheritance we can

provide for a child is freedom from the financial burden of caring for a parent.

MONEY AND CHILDREN

Parents may have problems talking about money. They wonder what and when to tell young children about the family's economic status. No parent wants an affluent child bragging about how much Daddy earns or a child in a struggling family worrying about Mommy losing her job.

In Boston where it was considered vulgar to talk about money, my parents never did ... except to clearly say "We can't afford it." when I asked for something beyond their means. However, somehow, money for education was always there. My years in medical school and my sister's years in college coincided. My parents somehow managed to provide the money we needed.

I answered a question from a mother who did not know how to divide assets in her will because one child's economic status was so much better than that of the siblings. I am not a lawyer and wills are a legal matter so I advised the mother to talk with a lawyer specializing in estate planning.

However, I do know lots about siblings and can tell you that twinges of sibling rivalry persist long into adulthood especially when money, property, or family heirlooms are involved. When wills are read, or when there is no will, sibling squabbles are almost inevitable. Even when the dollar amount is equally divided, if the Tiffany lamp that has been in the family for generations goes to the child who squeaked the loudest, things can get pretty ugly. And stay ugly.

Parents need to learn, as I did, the difference between "equal" and "equitable." Equal is defined mathematically; the dollar amount left to each child is the same. That is the easiest way to go. However, this is appropriate only if your children are all adults living independently on their own dime, are responsible about spending money, and have no physical or mental problems. Situations change so wills must be reviewed periodically.

Providing an equitable inheritance means each child gets what is fair after taking into account the needs of each child. A child with a disability may need lifelong support. One who is financially irresponsible or has an addiction may not be trusted to manage money. Lawyers will tell you a trust is the best way to deal with these problems. When parents gave a sizeable chunk of money to one child to start a business or buy a home, should they subtract that amount before dividing the estate? A tough decision. Best to discuss with a lawyer.

The most difficult issue to deal with, however, is what today's question raises, a glaring inequality between the children's incomes. One child decided on the arts instead of a profession or business and makes half of what the siblings earn. Or perhaps one child cannot get a job in his or her field because it is no longer needed. It is forecast that retail jobs may soon be nonexistent. Already since 2001, 18 times more department store workers than coal miners have lost their jobs.

My advice to parents is to gather all the children together to talk about this inequality. Remember the decision is yours to make and the will is yours to sign.

This family meeting is a good time to ask who wants what from the household effects. I have many of my artist mother's paintings and I asked my children to tell me which paintings they wanted. I recently took photos of my house and labeled them with information about every painting and family heirloom. I mailed these to all and again asked what each wanted. Only one conflict: my son had asked for the painting of a scarlet maple leaf years ago and my grandson just asked if he could have it. I'm still around so I could decide, guided by both seniority and the date of request. The painting will go to my son and my grandson picked out another picture.

My children, like many others, have different incomes. My late husband and I realized that we could not foresee the future ... an affluent child could be broke one day and another's status could improve. So we divided assets equally.

On the occasion of my husband's 80th birthday the family was gathered at a beautiful beach resort. At the birthday party, unbeknown to me, my husband handed each child an envelope with their name on it that contained a sizable check. He said he had been given a lifetime of presents and it was time to reverse the process. Confusion followed when the children opened the envelopes and realized each had each received another's check. My husband rose to tell all that he did this deliberately so they would remember handing money to a sibling and would always help each other out if necessary when he was gone. Nice!

A personal note. I ran a one-bed nursing home in our house for over three years when my husband developed dementia and needed care. Because he became much worse after a hospitalization, I felt he would do better at home and was able to do so. Hard on both the pocketbook and me. It was the hardest job I ever had.

When I was a child my father gently admonished me if I was on the road to do something I might regret. He would say "Marilyn, don't be foolish. Don't do anything foolish."

This advice is the perfect maxim for dealing with financial matters!

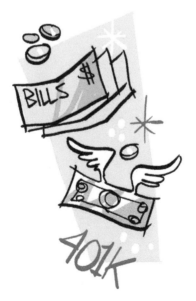

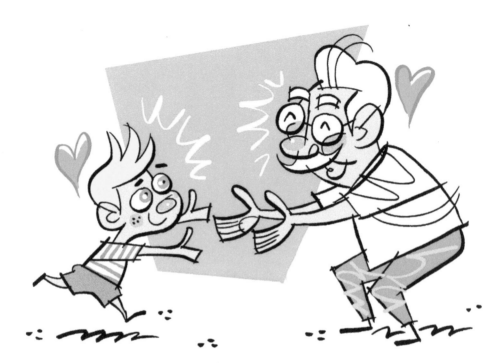

CHAPTER 22

GRANDPARENTING IN GERIATRICA

The happiest people I know in Geriatrica are those who have grandchildren living nearby. I define "living nearby" as being close enough so you can see a grandchild without having to get on an airplane.

There are a hefty 70 million of us grandparents now; our ranks are swelling with Baby Boomers.

Most residents of Geriatrica are already blessed with grandchildren. But, because some Geriatricians, me included, may have a memory lapse occasionally here is a short introduction to grandparenting.

GRANDPARENTING 101

Parenting advice changes like hemlines. But it is not just arbitrary fashion. Science propels our knowledge forward and guides us down safer pathways. Parenting also has changed. Many mothers are more educated, wait longer to have their first baby, and a higher percentage of mothers are in the workforce.

Lesson 1: The Importance of Grandparents.

When your grandchild is born you assume new roles. You are now a living ancestor, historian of the family and earlier times, teacher, mentor, helper, student of today's parenting, nurturer of baby and new mother, storyteller, crony, pal, playmate, wizard, hero, and role model on aging.

Lesson 2: What Grandparents Provide for their Grandchildren.

Unconditional love, stability, the important sense of family as well as identity and culture, knowledge both cognitive and practical, exposure to older people, exposure to your personal interests and skills, cushioning from hard knocks, courage, reinforcement of moral values, emotional and other support for the busy parents of their grandchildren.

Lesson 3: What Grandchildren Provide for Grandparents.

Fun! A grandchild is a great way to keep young and healthy. He or she provides an antidote to isolation and boredom, a sense of the future, connections to the world of the young, a way to stay current, a lesson in playfulness, a special and precious kind of love. A grandchild can be a wonderful pal. And at about age 12 he or she will be the perfect person to ask for help when your new digital gadget is misbehaving.

Lesson 4: The two big bad "I" words: Interference and Indulgence.

The best thing a grandmother can do for the mother of her new grandchild is trust New Mom to do a good job and increase confidence in her parenting skills. Choose your words carefully. Avoid criticism, praise lavishly, stay calm, be careful about your body language, and never check for dust on the bookshelves.

Before saying something that could be construed as criticism ask yourself 1) Will this help the mother of my grandbaby? 2) How would I have felt if my mother or mother-in-law said this to me?

However, if you think you could be helpful, say it right. "I notice you wash the kitchen floor every time you feed Liam in the high chair. I used to spread newspapers around the high chair and just rolled them up when the meal and throwing food was over." A wise woman I know told her daughter-in-law who was from another country, "Show me how you will care for your baby so I can help you the right way."

Humor helps. One grandmother of my acquaintance told her daughter-in-law, "I'm probably going to tell you what to do every minute but you don't have to listen!" Another wrote she was, "A 4-H grandma: Heart, Hugs, Help, and Hush up!"

Don't hush up helpful words said in a helpful way. "I know how you feel after a sleepless night. What can I do so you can take a nap?" Let compliments flow. Praise the new mother's loving care of the baby and her choice of nursery colors.

Respect New Mom's privacy and her need for self-time, time alone to bond with the baby, and time with the baby's father. Above all enjoy your relationship with her. Relish in the camaraderie that develops when two women bond over a baby. Love oozes!

You will indulge your grandchildren, we all do. But moderation in all things. Many, if not most, of American children suffer from Toy Overload. This disease causes the child to race from toy to toy not knowing where to start. It also leads to the "Gimme's" another disease that makes spoiled kids want even more toys. Toy Overload also has serious consequences for grandparental wallets. As a grandmother of twins, I can attest to that but what's a grandmother to do?

A word about Toy Overload. My daughter, the mother of twins whose toys overloaded the house, decided to set up a Toy Bank in a locked basement closet. In order to get out a toy, you had to put a toy back in the bank.

My favorite anecdote about grandchildren and presents: We flew to see a grandchild, age three, at Christmas time. His parents stayed up almost all night on Christmas Eve to put together a bright red car the child could get in and pedal. On Christmas morning he rushed to the car and pedaled it around the driveway with great glee. Soon tiring of this he came in the house and spent the whole day helping Grandpa make a house out of the huge carton the car came in. And then turning it into a garage filled with his miniature cars, then a zoo filled with little stuffed animals.

Grandparents, I don't want to take away all your fun. But today's toys tend to be noisy with lights that flash all over the place. Don't forget the old standbys like blocks especially when Grandpa or Grandma gets down on the floor to play. (One might have to stay vertical in case the other needs to be helped up!) The best toys are still those that foster imagination in children. Don't forget books!

Lesson 5: Sharing Your Story.

Here is a homework assignment for grandparents. It will take a little time and thought, but it will be fun and worthwhile for both you and your grandchildren.

Talk with your grandchildren whenever you can about yourself and your world. Remember that "talk with" includes listening and encouraging questions and comments.

Mostly we grandmas and grandpas talk to our grandkids about their world. How is school? What do you want to be when you grow up? Do you have a girlfriend or boyfriend yet? How's your job going?

Don't stop doing this but also talk about you and your world when you were growing up. The world changes so rapidly these days that we are "history" in the real sense of the word. Day-to-day life as we remember it does not make it into the history book. We know it well because we lived it.

What on earth does Dr. Heins expect me to say? This is the fun part: you say whatever you like. But keep it focused on **your** life as a child. Your first memory. Your first day at school. Favorite teacher. Dogs (or cats) in your childhood. Your best friend. Describe a typical day in say, sixth grade. Your first puppy love. Favorite subject in school. Favorite sport.

Your remembrances can coincide with the child's age or not. Your choice. Funny things that happened to you are always a hit. A child loves to hear about silly things grownup have done and if they should not have been done, you can add a sermon about why not to do such a thing.

Teens will like to hear about your adolescence, both the good parts and how you dealt with the painful parts. Nobody gets out of adolescence without some painful moments. But there are also wonderful moments and funny ones you can share.

Don't just talk about things or happenings. Talk about feelings. Something that made you happy. Something that made you sad. Something you wish you had not said or done. Things you worried about at different ages, especially dealing with things other kids said or did that were hurtful.

One thing that children love to hear about is what you did NOT have like color TV or cell phones. Think about what you have now that you didn't when you were the age of your grandchild. It's fun to chat with your grandkids about the changes and the speed of change. My grandchildren were astonished to hear that cars did not have seat belts when I was growing up. This led to us talking about auto safety.

One special tie to family history that we grandparents have is memories of our parents and other ancestors. Tell the grandchildren about your parents and grandparents. Get out the pictures of Great-Great-Grandfather standing next to his first car. And wedding pictures from the past. Clothes and hairdos may cause hilarity.

Think of yourself as the keeper of information about ancestors, everything including where they came from to the recipe for your grandmother's chicken soup. Over the last few years I have organized what information, photos, and family trees I had of ancestors on both sides of the family in separate files. I told my daughter who is my executor where they are kept so they can be passed on. Another file contains family recipes, the ones I both inherited and invented.

Do not think you have to do all this talking about your world at once. It's best to think about what would be both fun and useful to share. Jot your ideas down and bring then up at a quiet moment. When you and the grandchild are alone do not allow any distracting screens or other gadgets. Everyone paid rapt attention while the elders of yore told the oral history of our tribe.

Think of these special moments when historian grandparent and grandchild are together as your own serial story. BTW I kept my twin grandchildren spellbound with my own fictional serial of Mary McMotter, Girl Wizard (apologies to Harry). Every time we were together or had time to talk on the phone, I created another chapter on the spot. They all had the same theme: girl wizards count too. It's perfectly OK to include a bit of healthy propaganda in telling your story! As a matter of fact, it's a good idea.

CHILDREN OF GRANDPARENTS

Here is a job for you. Of course, you are busy raising the grandchildren. But keep an eye on your children's grandparents. As they age, they may not be as fit and able to visit you. They may suffer from Grandchild Deprivation Syndrome. This and Grandparent Deprivation Syndrome are serious, but curable with a little effort.

When our twin grandchildren were born on February 29, 1996, we were overjoyed. Boy-girl twins born on Leap Year Day who would not have their first birthday until the 21st century. Very special! We were there when they were born. I took each baby to the windows to introduce my two grandchildren to the world ... the sky, grass, trees.

My husband and I were determined to get to know, and be known, by these adorable bundles of joy. We flew more than halfway across the country every six to eight weeks. Left home on a Thursday and returned on Tuesday to accommodate our schedules.

We were able to watch the incredible growth and development of a child, one of the best shows on earth. It seems as though you can almost see the brain developing new connections!

Alas, even if one of these beloved twins produced triplets today, such multiple visits are not for this octogenarian. (I did go to the twins' graduations and I plan to stay alive to see my granddaughter graduate from medical school two years from now, even if I have to travel in a stretcher by ambulance plane!)

Recognizing that travel is hard for some seniors including Grandma, the twins fly here to visit me. They bring their significant others and we have a grand time. Obviously, grandparents and grandchildren are designed to have a grand time together! Between visits we text, call, and FaceTime ... not every day but enough to feel connected.

My daughter, son, daughter-in-law, and seven-year-old grandson just visited for my birthday. There is no better present on earth for a grandparent living in Geriatrica!

I had time to visit with each, a real treat!

My son reminded me, when he raised a glass to toast my age, that he once asked my mother on her birthday how it felt to be 95. She told him she still felt like a girl inside! I will check it out if I get there. At the present time I feel like a 50-year-old inside. I just remembered that one of my favorite nonagenarians loved to say, with a wicked gleam in her eye, "Oh, to be 70 again!"

WHAT I LEARNED FROM A SEVEN-YEAR-OLD

Seven-year-old Joshua, my youngest grandchild, is a joy to see in person. He raced to the pool first thing after hugging me. He had brought along a huge, inflatable beach ball. Transparent and covered with colorful dots, it still floats in our pool, blown by the wind, and proving that every reaction has an equal and opposite reaction as it hits the pool deck and sails off again and again.

We all dined out a couple of times. Grandma was delighted to see how civilized her grandchild was at a very grownup restaurant where he got his first taste of tiramisu and gave it a thumbs up. Joshua eats well and has some amazingly healthy choices like cucumber sticks or frozen blueberries for snacks. I now keep frozen blueberries in the freezer for those moments when I really want something cold and sweet that is not ice cream. The old and the young can learn from each other, right?

In addition to a hand-drawn birthday card from Joshua, I also was given a lesson in the life of elementary school kids today. I learned a lot.

Schoolchildren today are all taught what to do if there is an armed intruder in the school. When I was in school, we had fire drills. The bell meant we had to walk quickly but without running or pushing and take our designated exit route out of the building. These fire drills were always a surprise but were not scary, just a precaution we had to learn. A later generation of schoolkids were taught to duck and cover in case of a nuclear threat. I'm not sure if this scared them or not, but just thinking of it gives me the heebie-jeebies.

My daughter-in-law said Joshua's school does all it can to make this a routine drill like a fire drill ... something we have to do. I remember feeling very safe in elementary school and I knew the teachers would take care of me if anything happened. I feel awful thinking about second-graders like Joshua worrying about a gunman armed with a military weapon in his school.

I also learned that Lego bricks, the ones that were the same for years, have morphed. Now a Lego set has a theme and comes with tiny Lego figures of all sorts. Joshua showed me what they were and how he played with them.

He also showed me a gadget called Nintendo Switch, a video game you can play alone or take off the sides and play with another person. Very clever. He offered to teach me how to play but I declined. It would have been my first experience with a video game and I was scared. I watched him play alone and with his Mom. Just as I could never learn to play, let alone win, a game of poker in Las Vegas, this too is beyond me.

When I asked him, he assured me that video games were violent sometimes but it wasn't real, just a game. He has learned to download new games. He wins with glee and loses gracefully, if noisily. He also has a gadget at home that teaches simple computer programming and told me he would bring it next time so he could teach me how to do it. "It's easy, Grandma!"

I have been on the anti-video games side for a long time. I felt strongly that children should look at and interact with people not screens, games are violent, a waste of time, etc. But these games are part of Joshua's world.

Play in childhood has a vital purpose. It helps children learn not only skills, but also how the world works. Play is also a child's down time and everybody needs a break. My down time after homework and chores were done was reading ... my "drug" of choice was a book.

Joshua has an amazing schedule. School plus a full extracurricular life: karate, piano lessons, swimming (he was just advanced to the next level, came in fourth in his first race, and currently wants to be a famous swimming star like Michael Phelps), and cooking lessons.

He likes the outdoors and nature (has a bug palace), vanilla milkshakes, reading simple books on his own. He can amuse himself, and self-regulate. When he is tired or sulky, he goes to his room to read or play by himself. He does his chores (feeds the dogs and puts water in their bowls). He followed my directions to keep all his Lego pieces on one end of the table so we had room to eat.

Does he have no faults, doting Grandma? Of course he does. He is a noisy (hard on those of us with hearing aids) and pretty messy kid. But he wants and tries to please.

I learned a new trick that I share with other grandparents. To make sure that all the tiny Legos are accounted for, walk barefoot around the house! Your feet will find an amazing number of tiny plastic objects!

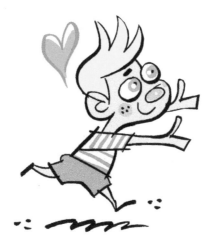

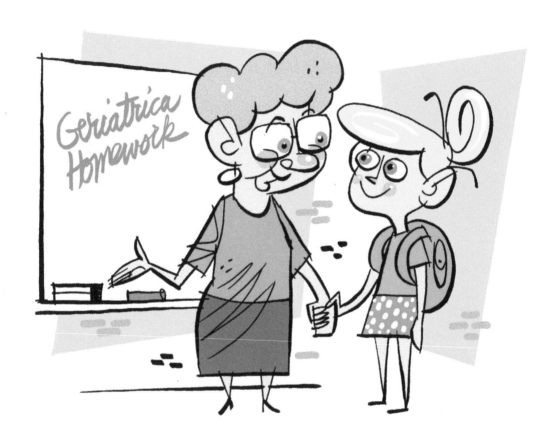

CHAPTER 23

TEACHING CHILDREN ABOUT GERIATRICA

Geriatrica is a land where we old people dwell. Children, who live in the Land of Youth, do not know much about our territory.

The two kindest and most loving statements I know are "Let me teach you." and "Let me help you."

We oldies in Geriatrica have a job to do. We are the only ones who can tell young children about aging and model how to be old. Let's teach the children what it is like to be old, as truthfully and cheerfully as we can.

Even very young grandchildren who visit us in Geriatrica can tell that we elderly people are different. We don't resemble the other grown-ups they know like parents and teachers. We may not move around easily the way younger adults do. We may have accoutrements like hearing aids, canes, walkers, portable oxygen. Visiting us in this new land can be scary at first.

I remember astonishment that my grandparents could take out their teeth! How funny that Grandma put her eyeglasses in the refrigerator and left the milk on the table! I was shushed and told it was not polite to laugh at other people even if the thing they did was funny.

Four-year-old me saw a grown man in a restaurant wearing a bib being fed by a woman. Like any little kid I pointed, giggled, and stared until my father told me to stop. "It's not polite to point and stare at people."

My own grandchild touched my flabby neck waving in the breeze and asked, "What's this, Grandma?" I told him the truth: "These are my wattles, Joshua." "Will I get them too?" "Not until you are very, very, very old."

Mr. Census Bureau tells me that the number of people age 65 and older is nearly 48 million, 14.9 percent of the total population. We are a big tribe.

But children today are often segregated from elderly people. We are a mobile society so a child's own grandparents may be thousands of miles away. Because people marry later and have children later, children may have either no grandparents or very elderly grandparents. Grandma is more likely to be in a retirement community than live in her child's house as in the past. Retirement communities, sadly, do not usually have children around.

A parent asked me about her child who did not want to visit her octogenarian grandfather.

"My son, 13, deals well with my often cranky and short-tempered father, now 80. My daughter is 11 and has expressed to me that she is not 'comfortable with old people.' My father is frail and doesn't make interesting conversation. Any hints on how to foster this relationship for as long as it is able to continue?"

I wrote, "I am really glad your daughter could express her feelings so clearly to you. Dealing with the frail elderly is difficult for many people as it requires lots of patience. The elderly can be slow in body movement and speech. What they do talk about can be very remote to an almost teen."

"Maybe your daughter can make her time with your father a sort of project. Suggest she tries to get Grandpa interested in what kids do these days like how you play a video game ? Reminisce with her about what your father was like when you were growing up. What were his accomplishments and interests? Maybe she could go over old photos with him to spark him up a bit.

"As long as she is attentive to your parent's needs (helps them up from a chair, gets them food from a buffet table) and treats them kindly, I would be satisfied for now. You don't want her to feel guilty when the inevitable happens."

For parents the challenge is to raise children who are sensitive to all kinds of people and who care about the feelings of others. This means your family values empathy, kindness, and helpfulness. You model these characteristics for your children and reward them with praise when they are exhibited.

Parents should make every effort to expose their children to us old guys. I attended my Aunt Helen's 90th birthday dinner in a Chinese restaurant in Boston. When the birthday cake was paraded through the room there was applause. Total strangers told her how wonderful she looked at 90 and one little girl asked for her autograph on a napkin!

No elderly people in your child's life? Adopt some. One family I know "adopted" an old gentleman from church. They asked him to share Sunday dinner every week and join the family for birthdays and other celebrations.

Invite elderly neighbors to holiday celebrations. Offer to drive them places. Bring your children with you when you help out an elderly neighbor. Children need to know what 90 looks like. And 90s thrive when they have contact with children!

GROWN-UP CHILDREN

We have one more task to do. We must teach our own grown children what it is like to be an elderly person living in Geriatrica. Some of us are aging well and look pretty good. Others, like the grandfather whose granddaughter avoided him, not so good.

When our children come to visit, we go all out to put our best foot forward. Sadly, in advanced old age, our best foot might be swollen or we are limping on it.

Grown children are never totally grown up. A part of them, the small child inside, wants their parents to stay around so they often see us in better shape than we are. Thus they can do well-meaning but inappropriate things.

"C'mon, Pop! I'll do the driving. All you have to do is sit there! It will be loads of fun! We'll go look at cars, stop at that restaurant you like and have a big bowl of chili you like so much!" When tired Pop gets home, he can hardly get out of the car fast enough to upchuck the chili that does not rest well in his old tummy. Pop has to learn to say no more long drives and chili.

Mom has to learn to say, "No, sorry I simply can't do Thanksgiving any more. But please come because we find holiday air travel tough these days. Either you guys shop and cook, or we order in, or we go out to eat." Mom also must learn to say, "We both need to rest sometime during the day, so you guys have to spend some time alone.

We have to politely say "No!" to our adult children just like when they were little kids. But instead of saying, "No, you must never do that again!" we have a new phrase, **"No, I can never do that again!"** It may feel funny at first but you will get used to it. And so will your children. If you taught them right!

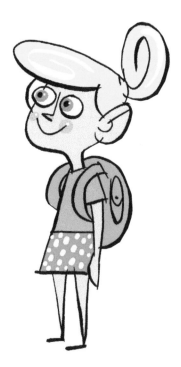

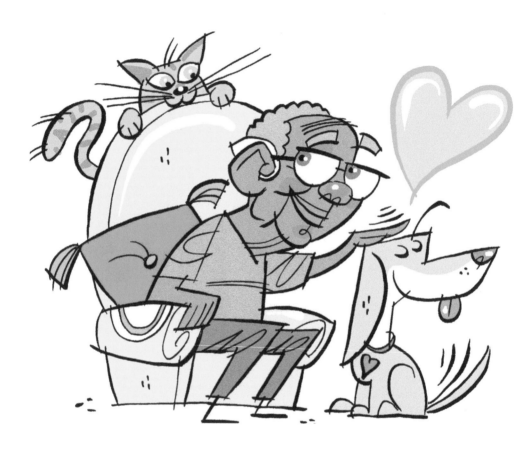

CHAPTER 24

CANINES WHO DWELL IN GERIATRICA

SHOULD ELDERFOLK GET A DOG?

Disclaimer: I write only about dogs because I have always had a dog. This is my pet of choice and always will be. My apologies to cat lovers!

Dog ownership is a big decision. You are inviting a living creature to live with you for the next 15 years or so if you choose a puppy. Issues to consider are SAFETY for both the owners and dog, WORK (who will care for Fido?) and EXPENSE.

SAFETY? Most diseases are species-specific (we have our viruses and dogs have theirs) but dogs can transmit certain skin conditions like ringworm and scabies. Regular checkups at the veterinarian keep both dog and human safe. Choosing the right dog in terms of size and breed and training the dog to behave can prevent bites.

WORK? Someone has to buy the food, feed the dog, clean up messes, train the dog, walk the dog, take the creature to the vet, etc. The pet will definitely add items to the EXPENSE side of your budget: food, toys, collars, licenses, pet door or cat box, veterinarian bills, neutering.

But there are many SPECIAL GIFTS a dog can bring. People get a very special type of unconditional love and affection from a dog. A canine creature makes eye contact, wags its tail, and is always ready to play. That's what distinguished them from wolves and why we have been feeding dogs for so many millennia!

Many dogs seem almost human in their ability to sense what a person is feeling. Years ago, I had just learned of the death of a dear one living far away and started crying. My Brittany Spaniel came over to me, put her head on my knee, and then reached up to lick the tears off my face.

What about the pros and cons of dogs for the elderly? In our age group ... roughly 65 to 105 ... dogs can be a positive and healthful addition to our lives. They can bring us friendship, purpose, and joy. They can even serve as canine "therapists" for those of us who are feeling lazy or blue.

Are they good therapists? According to Dr. Marwan Sabbagh of the Cleveland Clinic Center for Brain Health, "Simply petting an animal can decrease the level of the stress hormone cortisol and boost release of the neurotransmitter serotonin, resulting in lowered blood pressure and heart rate and, possibly, in elevated mood."

We are a herd mammal. The older we get the harder it is to herd. By circumstance or by choice, we find it difficult to get out and socialize. Those of us who are caregivers of a loved one can also be overwhelmed and isolated by their duties. We can all be cheered by the presence of a dog that exudes unconditional love.

Other pluses? I know from personal experience that a dog is the best "alarm clock" for a grieving or lazy oldie. Walking a dog may be the best exercise of all for us. It exercises both you and Fido. It almost guarantees social interaction both from fellow dog-walkers and solo neighbors.

As the Cleveland Clinic suggests, "Get your six legs out there!" Walking a dog not only provides you with exercise but can even help your brain keep healthy.

Therapy and Service dogs can also be of great help to those of us in Geriatrica with specific needs.

It is essential that you: 1) Pick your dog carefully. An orthopedic surgeon I know points out that big dogs and exuberant, poorly leash-trained small dogs can cause the dog-owner to fall and fracture a bone. Bad for anybody especially those in Geriatrica. 2) Train the dog well yourself or, if that is not possible, have the dog professionally trained to walk on leash and not lunge, for your own safety.

Getting an older dog with a good temperament from an animal shelter can be perfect. It benefits **two** species, human and canine, at the same time!

Think realistically. It is important to protect your dog from ending up in an animal shelter when you are no longer able to care for it or are not around anymore. I arranged with my daughter, also my executor and a dog owner and dog lover, to care for the dog I acquired if I could not longer do so.

For spouses and children of an elderly person, listen up! My veterinarian husband pointed out that using a dog as a Christmas or birthday present is not always a good idea. It's like an arranged marriage in a tribe of humans that pick their own mates. Be sure your gift will be appropriate and appreciated before you shop.

A PERSONAL DOG TALE

Let me tell you a dog tail, sorry I mean tale.

Once upon a time three old creatures inhabited our house, two humans and one canine.

Old human creatures have a commonality…they are no longer young. Body parts are wearing out, some at an accelerated pace. Activities start to decrease. We begin to have "Thoughts of when I cease to be … " (I just looked up the Keats poem to check on my memory and he actually wrote "fears" not "thoughts." I had made a sort of optimistic memory mistake.)

All three of us, both human and canine, have health "issues" the delicate way to describe the effects of having decrepit body parts. We all take a bunch of pills each day and we see our doctor as required or requested. We all have plumbing problems and decreasing stamina.

But we three get up and take our walk together every morning. We upright ones cherish our mobility and want to keep it as long as possible. I consider it a victory every time I can bend down to gather Mindy's poop in the dog waste bag. And straighten up again!

At this point in time the sickest of the three creatures is the dog. My beloved Cavalier King Charles Spaniel came to live with me 13 years ago.

My late husband had made it clear that he did not want another dog after his beloved Brittany Spaniel died. As he became sicker, I felt I needed a dog. My niece arranged for Mindy to be shipped to me from Texas as Mindy was perfect for me. She had been living with the breeder who had hoped to show her but she did not weigh enough to be shown. She was six months old and trained.

I had concocted a fib that the dog was for my niece, if objections were raised. When I brought Mindy into the house, my husband asked, "Whose dog is this?" as Mindy gently jumped into his lap and kissed him. "Ours if you like her." "Like her? I love her!"

The feeling was mutual. When my husband, on home hospice care became bedridden, she jumped onto his bed and kept a canine vigil. When he died, she licked my tears.

Mindy has enriched my life from the moment I picked her up at the airport. In my arms for the first time she tremblingly whimpered and kissed my face after her ordeal in the crate. Loud noise and a sensation of falling will make every baby fearful. Puppies too, but they stop whimpering to kiss you.

Mindy adjusted quickly and completely to her new house and owners. She commandeered her own place on the sofa and on the bed. She knew where the treats were kept and would stand there looking up hopefully. She outgrew her chew toys in favor of playing Red Dot, chasing a laser pointer down the hall and through the house. This talented King Charles Spaniel even wrote me a poem:

> I'm the King of the Castle
> And at the top of the hill,

I drop my royal pooplets
To give my subjects a thrill!

The lady I live with who walks me
Always picks them up,
Lest the neighbors think
I'm just a common pup.

I feel like a royal canine
And I always look the part,
And love keeps overflowing
From my royal heart!

Sadly, royal Mindy developed congestive heart failure, a common problem in this breed. She actually takes more pills than I do (and old dogs do not have Medicare Part D).

Her symptoms have been helped by medication but her veterinarian has gently told me she cannot be cured. We realize she is on a downhill course. Would you know it if you saw her today? No. Every morning she eagerly wags her tail in greeting when I open the curtains to watch the first finches arrive at the feeder outside the window.

Mindy takes her medicine as prescribed. One pill is chewable and she considers it a treat. I dip a wooden coffee stirrer into the peanut butter jar to get a small dab that the other pills stick to. Mindy eagerly swallows the pill-studded dab and then positions the end of the wooden stick so her teeth scrape up every molecule of peanut butter!

She knows the route we walk by heart and tugs the leash to sniff each favorite rock and bush. Some days she is frisky, other days she walks more slowly. She still plays Red Dot but doesn't run as fast or as long as other days. She chews more slowly and has to peer to find a morsel of people food that falls on the floor ... she formerly would pounce on in a nano-second. She is forgetful but who cares about the occasional diuretic-induced accident on the carpet? We don't.

Now she sleeps much of the day. Because she is deaf (like me without my hearing aids) when she is asleep I must approach her very gently or she startles anxiously until she realizes who it is. She skips an occasional meal but is always eager to get an occasional treat that both humans are just as eager to provide.

All she worries about is that we come back when we leave the house. Her love of us is profound, deep, and unconditional. She doesn't know we are old so she doesn't fret about losing us.

We watched "Victoria" on PBS. Queen Victoria was given a King Charles Spaniel named Dash when she was 13. TV showed the young Queen coming back to her chambers from a royal event to find Dash stretched out dead on the floor. This is factual, the dog died at age 10 and was buried by the Queen herself. When I saw the dead dog (who looked like Mindy's twin) tears rolled down my cheeks.

But after drying my eyes and on reflection, what better way for a beloved dog to die? At home when the owner is not around to rush her to the veterinarian. Never placed in a doggie ICU. Best of all sparing me from the ordeal of deciding Mindy no longer can live a quality dog life so I must now take her on that last sad trip to the veterinarian.

We humans understand the concept of a future and of death. Almost every one I know says they do not fear death, rather they fear loss of independence, autonomy, mobility, brain function.

Mindy does not. She assumes we will always care for her and love her. And we will.

ELEGY FOR MINDY

My beloved Mindy, was born November 15, 2005, and died June 8, 2018. May she rest in peace in doggie heaven.

A condolence email from a friend: "I always wonder about a new pet when I know how hard the end will be. But the great quantities of joy that our little doggie brings is immeasurable."

Memories of all Mindy did for me abound. She saved my life by getting me out of bed each morning after my husband died when all I wanted to do was crawl deep under the covers and stay there. She brought me much joy every day during our precious time together. And when she developed congestive heart failure, she bore her infirmity and took her medicine with royal grace as befits a Cavalier King Charles Spaniel.

But her infirmities worsened and increased. Mindy became totally deaf. She was getting lame and could no longer jump on the bed or sofa so was relegated to the floor unless we lifted her up. She began to refuse to walk, slept most of the time, and even had problems chewing her dog food. Her rotting teeth needed attention but because of her heart condition she could not be given anesthesia. Sometimes she seemed out of it, like she had doggie Alzheimer's.

Our loving care for her included making a painful decision. The last three weeks of her life were very difficult. In addition to her heart failure her gastrointestinal system was acting up. She began to refuse food and developed intractable diarrhea. Treatments we tried didn't work. She lost almost two pounds from a peak weight of 13. She started vomiting all food and starving to death was an unthinkable end.

Mindy's trusted veterinarian listened to my account of her condition. He said we could try heroic treatments but in her overall condition they were unlikely to work. We agreed the quality of her life was horrible. But when she was in my arms and we made eye contact her tail wagged, albeit feebly. What would she want?

My decision, which I feel was the right one, was painfully difficult. Heavy-hearted I made the decision to euthanize her and signed the writ of execution. She was sedated and fell asleep in my lap. Her end was peaceful and humane. I asked for cremation and scattered her ashes along her favorite walk. I was sent a condolence card signed by all those who worked at the veterinary hospital and also received a ceramic footprint of Mindy's paw.

I confess that as a woman in advanced old age, I had a twinge of jealousy. When our end is certain and hopeless most of us do not have the humane option Mindy had ... although some states have or are looking into assisted suicide. (Humans do, however, have superb hospice and palliative care available, two humane medical programs that relieve suffering.)

We humans, blessed with the ability to understand a future and plan for our aging, must make end of life decisions for ourselves and our spouse. Planning for our own end of life is prudent. (See Chapter 21.)

I am sure Mindy, who loved her human family as much as we loved her, would understand and approve.

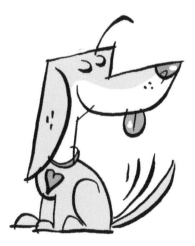

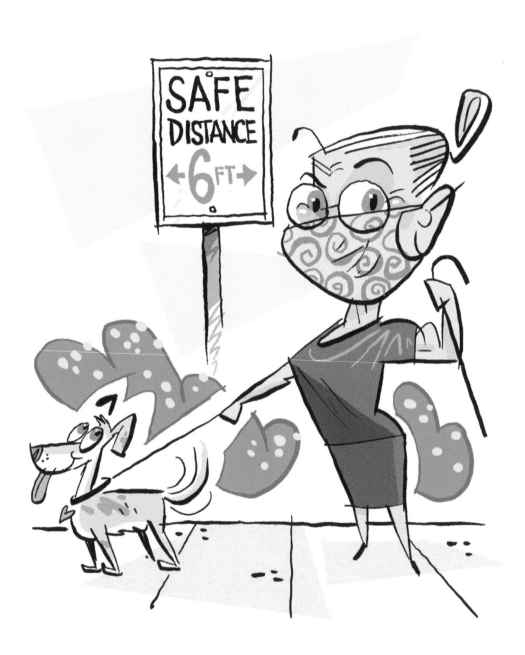

CHAPTER 25

COVID-19 INVADES GERIATRICA!

OUR PERSONAL STORY

On Friday, March 15, 2020, we were already downsized, the movers were hired, and colorful stickers dotted many objects in the house telling the movers what to put where in our new apartment. We had a moving date and were ready to go.

But it was not to be. A call from Hacienda at the Canyon, the brand-new independent living community we were scheduled to move into, changed everything. Because of the Great Pandemic of 2020, new residents are not allowed to move in until it becomes safe to do so. As of this writing we are still banned.

Hacienda is a spacious senior community with many amenities designed to foster interaction. We were seeking the exact opposite of what we have now. We longed for social interaction, not social distancing!

We are in a coronavirus "vulnerable group" because of our age and pre-existing medical conditions. At present we live in a single home on a quiet street. We are pretty active for our age (me, 90; him, 98). As the number of cases began to increase, we decided to ensure our social distancing by not leaving our home at all except for doctor's appointments where we are dutifully masked. Food is delivered.

We still take our daily morning walk and pay attention to the friendly neighborhood dogs who greet us while keeping a "social distance" from their owners. We have counted our pills, tallied our food, and are hoping for the best.

Still, there is much sad emptiness in our lives. Relatives and friends postponed visits. Calendars were wiped clean by cancellations everywhere … concerts, classes, restaurant dates, the MetHD opera. Looking at blank page after page in my Weekly Appointment Book (an admittedly archaic way of keeping track of one's life) is actually startling. I confess to sometimes not knowing what day it is when I wake up. Senility? Stress? I prefer to blame the latter and there is some evidence for that.

That Brain Fog You're feeling is Perfectly Normal by neuropsychologist Molly Colvin makes some reassuring points. When we are confronted with danger, we react physiologically to prepare our body for "fight or flight." There are also cognitive changes. We focus hard on the threat and, from an evolutionary perspective, this focus was vital when a wild animal crossed our path. "Complex thinking skills, like decision-making or planning, temporarily go offline," says Dr. Colvin."

Alas when we are dealing with chronic stress especially when there are multiple stressors…the pandemic, police brutality and pervasive racism, uncertainty about our physical or financial future, worry about our kids and grandkids … these cognitive changes may become worrisome.

I notice my own pesky cognitive changes. It is sometimes hard to focus or make decisions. Tasks take longer, mistakes are made. I am more forgetful than usual. Of course, this makes me cross with myself.

Dr. Colvin explains, "Frustrating as it may be, brain fog may actually be protective." It helps us focus on safety and prevents cognative overlaod so we can focus on new skills.

My first new skill was learning how to deal with the effects of brain fog. I try to distract myself in pleasant and healthy ways, be kind to myself and others, forgive myself my brain lapses and irritability, and do my exercises.

My man is more mellow than I am. He accepts the way things are because "I can't do anything about it." True. But inside of this old me there is still a residue of that younger me who wants to fix things. Because I can't make the virus go away, I feel helpless and anxious. I, like everybody else, live in uncertainty that leads to anxiety.

We are together, as healthy as two really old geezers can be, and have a roof over our heads. Everybody's world all over the world has changed and none of us know how, when, or whether we will get it back. Each of us is now living with fear, indecision, uncertainty, and no clear sense of when the crisis will be over. Also, alas, our house is super-fragilistic-discombobulated from our downsizing efforts.

My advice to myself and my readers is to search within to find some equanimity. Help others do the same by staying in virtual touch with each other. Be grateful we have telephones, email, video chat, FaceTime, and social media through which portals we can stay in touch, comfort each other, and get through this unbelievable but real crisis together even though we are apart.

Hope for the future and a positive outlook is healthy. Laughter is healthy. I called out to my pool lady, "I hope you washed your hands before you dared touch my pool." We had a good laugh together when she pointed out her hands were the cleanest in town ... they were in chlorine all day long!

MY BIG, FAT WORRIES

First, the virus! I am adapting to the unimaginable current situation, or trying to. I realize that everybody is affected in some way and that many or most have it a lot worse than I do. Yet my list of places and things that I miss and hope will come back quick continues to lengthen. I miss my friends and family more, not less, every day. I long for that date in the future when the pandemic ends because I really miss maskless faces, face-to-face conversation, hugs, and handshakes.

Second, I am very upset that systemic racism and police hyper-militarism seems to be part of America's DNA. The riots and protests that fill our TV screens and newspapers are troubling to see, though the continued protest is heartwarming. The political situation is unbelievable and scary. We are NOT one nation indivisible … we are in partisanship hell. Much must be done but it is too close to stalemate from my point of view.

I remember a very much earlier race riot when a just turned six-year-old boy asked his mom, "What's a Negro? Have I ever seen one?" The startled mother said, "Jimmy was at your birthday party!" The little boy said, "Is Jimmy a Negro? I didn't know that!"

Children have to be taught to hate as the masterful lyrics from the Rodgers and Hammerstein musical *South Pacific* tell us:

"You've got to be taught before it's too late,

Before you are six or seven or eight,

To hate all the people your relatives hate,

You've got to be carefully taught!"

Listen up parents, grandparents, and teachers. We have an enormous task ahead. All children must be taught about the evils of slavery and how NOT to hate! The message from every person and pulpit is simple. We are one people on a fragile planet and we must work together. Everybody is needed to change our course.

My third worry? The first Terrible Wildfire of 2020. I live in the foothills of Tucson's Catalina Mountains. We saw a ring of fire as spectacular as the one in *Valkyrie* for the Wagner fans out there. At night the visible fire seemed to be only one mountain ridge away from our house. We asked close neighbors what they thought. Both said they were staying in place for now, as did we.

However, the next morning we realized that our home was only two streets away from the area now designated Set, the second of the three safety stages: Ready, Set, Go! Because we had a house available that was not in the fire path, we grabbed essentials and went.

We were safe, comfortable and cool with ample food and reading material.

I admit I suffer from the psychological effects of three plagues piling on me all at once. How strange that a new virus, massive racial unrest, and a raging wildfire melded together in time.

Readers: I admit to being worried about all three of these plagues. The worry area of my brain was definitely overloaded.

I played a little game with my thoughts. On the drive to the safe house, I pretended I was going to a beautiful resort on a tropical beach. Usually when I get out of the shower, I turn off the ceiling fan but at the resort I just pretended it was a sea breeze! (My psychiatrist daughter assures me it's OK to pretend, just don't dive into the driveway pretending it's an ocean!)

UNCERTAINTY

Uncertainty stalks us. Even the best TV or print punditry does not provide or foster certainty. We miss our old routines but keeping old routines is impossible. Try to make your life and your family's lives as predictable as you can. I summon up courage by reminding myself the lack of predictability is worldwide. I try to cheer up my down friends on the phone or via computer messages. They reciprocate, bless them.

ADVICE TO WE THE OLD PEOPLE

This advice for the elderly population comes from an Official Old Lady. Our lives have has been changed by social distancing. We are stuck at home. It may be tempting to do away with our predictable routines.

Not a good idea but you can tweak them a bit. Sleep later if you like, but do not stay in pajamas all day, at least not too often. Not good for the soul. Eat regular healthy meals but once in a while have a gooey goodie. Go through the motions of your usual cleaning schedule. Have or find a hobby. Use this time to improve skills or learn something new. When all else fails you can always clean the garage, organize photos, or write a book!

Keep in touch with family and friends every way you can. Send a handwritten letter just for the fun and novelty of it. I make an effort every day to call a bunch of friends for socialize-by-ear sessions. Virtual contact is better than none, so I do lots of emailing not only to submit my columns and order food but also to socialize with dear ones far away. I also Facetime and Zoom.

REMEMBER THE CHILDREN

Abigail Adams told her president husband John Adams to remember the ladies. Dr. Heins is telling you to remember the children. This is awfully tough on them. No school, no play, worried parents, no visits from Grandma even on a birthday.

We all worry about our children and grandchildren. Here are some ParenTips:

BE HONEST.

EXPRESS YOUR OWN FEELINGS.

SAY YOU WILL DO EVERYTHING IN YOUR POWER TO KEEP THE FAMILY SAFE.

ENCOURAGE YOUR CHILD TO TALK ABOUT WHAT IS HAPPENING.

LEARN ABOUT VIRUSES TOGETHER (How they are named, why they spread worldwide so quickly, what immunity is, how vaccines are made, why social distancing and masks are so important.).

INVOLVE CHILDREN IN FAMILY PROJECTS.

GIVE LOTS OF HUGS. Have a family hug three times a day like meals.

LIMIT TV.

UTILIZE NATURE, OUR UNIVERSAL HEALER. Spend socially distanced time out of doors.

STRUCTURE THE DAY.

HANG IN THERE TOGETHER! Picture your child or grandchild in the future saying to the grandchildren of the future, "Let me tell you about the Great Pandemic of 2020!"

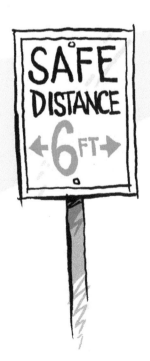

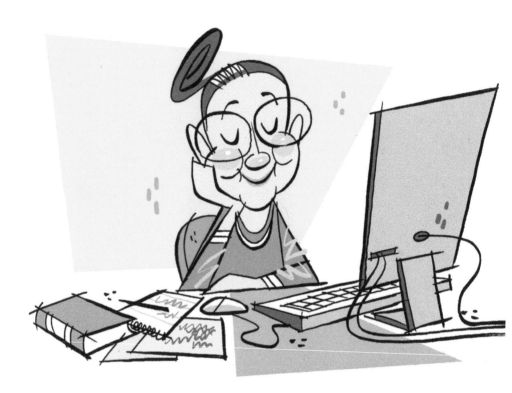

CHAPTER 26

CODA

The term coda is an Italian word that means tail. It is used at the end of a musical work to sort of sum up the notes and phrases of the piece.

This is my coda, the end of my book.

I hope my words have been helpful and that the Fitzsimmons drawings have lifted your spirits.

I also hope this book has not been a downer for you. Some things about aging and life in Geriatrica are serious and downright painful to think about.

A friend once asked me this question. "You write about hassles in your life, things you don't like about the world or about aging. Why don't you tell us about what you do like about your life and being old?"

How do I love my life in Geriatrica? Let me count the ways! I love poetry so it is fitting that I paraphrase poet Elizabeth Barrett Browning.

I love that I am still here. Yes, aging means there are more aches and pains, an increasing number and severity of medical problems, more trials and tribulations. I have worries about my own old age and that of those I care about. I worry about my country and the planet. But even on really bad days, I try to find things in my life or surroundings to appreciate and love.

One of the best things about aging is that, despite the losses, most of us retain a long lifetime of memories. I catch the glimpse of a child's photograph and cannot help smiling. I see a crooked ceramic bowl made for me by a schoolchild nearly 50 years ago and feel as proud as I did then. A friend's phone call or witty email lifts my spirits.

I love the outdoor landscape. I lived at sea level until I moved to Tucson 40 years ago. In my sea level days I loved standing on the shore of the Atlantic Ocean or a great lake to see the vast horizon. I still love the ocean and walking along a beach but I fell in love with the mountains surrounding the Tucson valley. My husband called the Catalinas "Marilyn's Mountains" because of all my oo-ing and ah-ing.

My favorite things out of doors? The glorious sunsets, clouds, saguaros, the spring burst of yellow, the birds and birdsongs. Also the fascinating wild creatures I see in my yard or on my walk ... from baby bunnies to coyotes, from spade-footed toads to Gila monsters.

Indoors? I love reading a new book, especially literary fiction, and also old favorites including my annual reread of *Little Women*. Music, live classical music, is my cultural drug of choice. My favorites in alphabetical order are Arizona Friends of Chamber Music, True Concord, and the Tucson Symphony Orchestra plus opera both live at Arizona Opera and at the Metropolitan Opera Live in HD in a movie theater.

Cinema has been a passion of mine since I lived in Manhattan and could see old and foreign movies free on Saturdays at The Museum of Modern Art. I love a good movie at the Loft Cinema. But on tired days I love that we can stream at home.

I am addicted to taking courses at the Humanities Seminars Program at the University of Arizona (I have taken well over 60 of them) to feed my still insatiable curiosity. And I love what I am doing right now, writing!

I am grateful for my loving family and the man I love. I am the last of my generation except for two cousins. I have two children, two stepsons, two daughters-in-law, one son-in-law, five grandchildren, and two young great-grandsons to love and watch grow in height and life knowledge.

My many friends enrich my life. I have lost several friends

recently and miss them greatly. But I am grateful for their memory.

I thank goodness for my mobility, creaky as it is. Yes my joints ache especially the knees and neck but I push myself to walk every day. I do balance exercises so I can avoid falls (fingers crossed) and maintain being mobile.

I can still see and hear albeit with assistance. My skin, marred by bruises upon bruises, and hair are both thinning at a now rapid rate. I told my dermatologist that I hoped my skin would last as long as I did. She told me it usually works out that way.

I can still drive. However unlike many elders I know, I am willing to relinquish this when I feel it is not safe just as I decided to give up hiking when I reached 80 and stepping on a ladder or even a lowly step stool when I reached 85.

I try to love the attributes I have retained more than regret those I have lost. I am grateful for my curiosity. Curiosity starts at birth when the baby seeks and finds its mother's face. All our lives we try to make sense of our world and ourselves. I still love to learn new things and make connections to what I already know ... even if I forget some of them!

I love to laugh, especially after I have been grumpy or sullen. I love to see generosity, friendship, and respect for others ... especially in today's crazy world.

I love getting emails from friends who share both their knowledge and wisdom. One example, when writing about aging, "We should copy the canines. Elderly dogs accept their aging and limitations with courage and grace. They sleep a lot, never complain, and seem to be enveloped in a calm peace, evidence of a life well lived." I agree and hope all of us can reach the end of our lives thusly!

As part of getting my affairs in order as they say (I smile at the phrase and confess to my readers I was too busy to have any affairs!) I wrote the following directions for my memorial service to the executor of my estate. (I never had a manorial estate either!)

Please read the following passage written by W.N.P. Barbellion, pen name of Bruce Cummings (1889-1919), British diarist who died young of Multiple Sclerosis.

I came across this in a book by David Lodge called *Deaf Sentence*. I was at one of my several book groups (I love book groups too!) when I realized that this quote exactly expresses my feelings about life and death. It is an "honour" and a privilege and a pleasure to live and love.

It was while I was writing this, that I noticed that Bruce Cummings and I were both born on September 7, a heart-thumping coincidence!

"To me the honour is sufficient of belonging to the universe—such a great universe, and so grand a scheme of things. Not even Death can rob me of that "honour". For nothing can alter the fact that I have lived; I have been I, if for ever so short a time and when I am dead the matter which composes my body is indestructible—and eternal, so that come what may to my 'soul,' my dust will always be going on, each separate atom of me playing its separate part—I shall still have some sort of finger in the pie. When I am dead, you can boil me, burn me, drown me, scatter me—but you cannot destroy me: my little atoms would merely deride such heavy vengeance. Death can do no more than kill you."

Am I frightened of what is to come? Absolutely, not of death but of a lingering, debilitating illness. I know I am on the downward trajectory of aging and there is only one way to get off the ramp. But why dwell on sad thoughts? I try instead to focus on being happy to be alive. Look the sun has risen on another day! Lucky me!

My sister used to say that life was made up of good moments and bad moments and we should all hope to get our share of good moments. Although her death was one of my worst moments, I have had a bounteous share of good moments.

FINIS! I made it!

CPSIA information can be obtained
at www.ICGtesting.com
Printed in the USA
LVHW022210251120
672563LV00013B/392